Application of Retinal and Optic Nerve Imaging in Clinical Medicine 2.0

Application of Retinal and Optic Nerve Imaging in Clinical Medicine 2.0

Editors

Rodolfo Mastropasqua
Rossella D'Aloisio

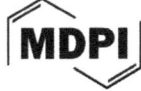

Basel • Beijing • Wuhan • Barcelona • Belgrade • Novi Sad • Cluj • Manchester

Editors
Rodolfo Mastropasqua
Ophthalmology Clinic,
Department of Neuroscience,
Imaging and Clinical Sciences
University G. D'Annunzio
Chieti-Pescara
Chieti, Italy

Rossella D'Aloisio
Ophthalmology Clinic,
Department of Medicine and
Science of Ageing
University G. D'Annunzio
Chieti-Pescara
Chieti, Italy

Editorial Office
MDPI
St. Alban-Anlage 66
4052 Basel, Switzerland

This is a reprint of articles from the Special Issue published online in the open access journal *Journal of Clinical Medicine* (ISSN 2077-0383) (available at: https://www.mdpi.com/journal/jcm/special_issues/Retinal_Optic_Nerve).

For citation purposes, cite each article independently as indicated on the article page online and as indicated below:

Lastname, A.A.; Lastname, B.B. Article Title. *Journal Name* **Year**, *Volume Number*, Page Range.

ISBN 978-3-0365-9180-3 (Hbk)
ISBN 978-3-0365-9181-0 (PDF)
doi.org/10.3390/books978-3-0365-9181-0

© 2023 by the authors. Articles in this book are Open Access and distributed under the Creative Commons Attribution (CC BY) license. The book as a whole is distributed by MDPI under the terms and conditions of the Creative Commons Attribution-NonCommercial-NoDerivs (CC BY-NC-ND) license.

Contents

Jose Javier Garcia-Medina, Nieves Bascuñana-Mas, Paloma Sobrado-Calvo,
Celia Gomez-Molina, Elena Rubio-Velazquez, Maravillas De-Paco-Matallana, et al.
Macular Anatomy Differs in Dyslexic Subjects
Reprinted from: *J. Clin. Med.* **2023**, *12*, 2356, doi:10.3390/jcm12062356 1

Raphael Diener, Jost Lennart Lauermann, Nicole Eter and Maximilian Treder
Discriminating Healthy Optic Discs and Visible Optic Disc Drusen on Fundus Autofluorescence
and Color Fundus Photography Using Deep Learning—A Pilot Study
Reprinted from: *J. Clin. Med.* **2023**, *12*, 1951, doi:10.3390/jcm12051951 13

Filippo Tatti, Claudio Iovino, Giuseppe Demarinis, Emanuele Siotto Pintor,
Marco Pellegrini, Oliver Beale, et al.
En Face Choroidal Vascularity in Both Eyes of Patients with Unilateral Central Serous
Chorioretinopathy
Reprinted from: *J. Clin. Med.* **2023**, *12*, 150, doi:10.3390/jcm12010150 23

Marco Rocco Pastore, Serena Milan, Rossella Agolini, Leonardo Egidi, Tiziano Agostini,
Lorenzo Belfanti, et al.
How Could Medical and Surgical Treatment Affect the Quality of Life in Glaucoma Patients?
A Cross-Sectional Study
Reprinted from: *J. Clin. Med.* **2022**, *11*, 7301, doi:10.3390/jcm11247301 33

Livio Vitiello, Maddalena De Bernardo, Luca Erra, Federico Della Rocca, Nicola Rosa and
Carolina Ciacci
Optical Coherence Tomography Analysis of Retinal Layers in Celiac Disease
Reprinted from: *J. Clin. Med.* **2022**, *11*, 4727, doi:10.3390/jcm11164727 45

Olimpia Guarino, Claudio Iovino, Valentina Di Iorio, Andrea Rosolia, Irene Schiavetti,
Michele Lanza and Francesca Simonelli
Anatomical and Functional Effects of Oral Administration of Curcuma Longa and Boswellia
Serrata Combination in Patients with Treatment-Naïve Diabetic Macular Edema
Reprinted from: *J. Clin. Med.* **2022**, *11*, 4451, doi:10.3390/jcm11154451 55

Rossella D'Aloisio, Matteo Gironi, Tommaso Verdina, Chiara Vivarelli, Riccardo Leonelli,
Cesare Mariotti, et al.
Early Structural and Vascular Changes after Within-24 Hours Vitrectomy for Recent Onset
Rhegmatogenous Retinal Detachment Treatment: A Pilot Study Comparing Bisected Macula
and Not Bisected Macula
Reprinted from: *J. Clin. Med.* **2022**, *11*, 3498, doi:10.3390/jcm11123498 63

Claudio Iovino, Clemente Maria Iodice, Danila Pisani, Luciana Damiano, Valentina Di Iorio,
Francesco Testa and Francesca Simonelli
Clinical Applications of Optical Coherence Tomography Angiography in Inherited Retinal
Diseases: An Up-to-Date Review of the Literature
Reprinted from: *J. Clin. Med.* **2023**, *12*, 3170, doi:10.3390/jcm12093170 77

Jo-Hsuan Wu and Tin Yan Alvin Liu
Application of Deep Learning to Retinal-Image-Based Oculomics for Evaluation of Systemic
Health: A Review
Reprinted from: *J. Clin. Med.* **2023**, *12*, 152, doi:10.3390/jcm12010152 91

Matteo Gironi, Rossella D'Aloisio, Tommaso Verdina, Benjamin Shkurko, Lisa Toto and Rodolfo Mastropasqua
Bilateral Branch Retinal Vein Occlusion after mRNA-SARS-CoV-2 Booster Dose Vaccination
Reprinted from: *J. Clin. Med.* **2023**, *12*, 1325, doi:10.3390/jcm12041325 . . . . **101**

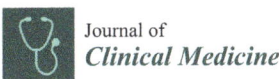

Article

Macular Anatomy Differs in Dyslexic Subjects

Jose Javier Garcia-Medina [1,2,3,4,5,6,*], Nieves Bascuñana-Mas [2], Paloma Sobrado-Calvo [1,2,5,6], Celia Gomez-Molina [2,3], Elena Rubio-Velazquez [3], Maravillas De-Paco-Matallana [3], Vicente Zanon-Moreno [4,5,6,7], Maria Dolores Pinazo-Duran [4,5,6,8,†] and Monica Del-Rio-Vellosillo [9,10,†]

1. Department of Ophthalmology, Optometry, Otorhinolaryngology and Pathology, University of Murcia, 30100 Murcia, Spain
2. General University Hospital Reina Sofia, 30003 Murcia, Spain
3. General University Hospital Morales Meseguer, 30008 Murcia, Spain
4. Ophthalmic Research Unit "Santiago Grisolia", 46017 Valencia, Spain
5. Spanish Net of Ophthalmic Pathology OFTARED RD16/0008/0022, Institute of Health Carlos III, 28029 Madrid, Spain
6. Spanish Net of Inflammatory Diseases RICORS, Institute of Health Carlos III, 28029 Madrid, Spain
7. Faculty of Health Sciences, International University of Valencia, 46002 Valencia, Spain
8. Cellular and Molecular Ophthalmobiology Group, Surgery Department, Faculty of Medicine and Odontology, University of Valencia, 46010 Valencia, Spain
9. University Hospital Virgen de la Arrixaca, 30120 Murcia, Spain
10. Department of Surgery, Obstetrics and Gynecology and Pediatrics, University of Murcia, 30100 Murcia, Spain
* Correspondence: jj.garciamedina@um.es
† Monica del-Rio-Vellosillo and Maria Dolores Pinazo-Duran share the last authorship as senior authors.

Abstract: The macula, as the central part of the retina, plays an important role in the reading process. However, its morphology has not been previously studied in the context of dyslexia. In this research, we compared the thickness of the fovea, parafovea and perifovea between dyslexic subjects and normal controls, in 11 retinal segmentations obtained by optical coherence tomography (OCT). With this aim, we considered the nine sectors of the Early Treatment Diabetic Retinopathy Study (ETDRS) grid and also summarized data from sectors into inner ring subfield (parafovea) and outer ring subfield (perifovea). The thickness in all the four parafoveal sectors was significantly thicker in the complete retina, inner retina and middle retina of both eyes in the dyslexic group, as well as other macular sectors (fovea and perifovea) in the inner nuclear layer (INL), inner plexiform layer (IPL), IPL + INL and outer plexiform layer + outer nuclear layer (OPL + ONL). Additionally, the inner ring subfield (parafovea), but not the outer ring subfield (perifovea), was thicker in the complete retina, inner retina, middle retina (INL + OPL + ONL), OPL + ONL, IPL + INL and INL in the dyslexic group for both eyes. In contrast, no differences were found between the groups in any of the sectors or subfields of the outer retina, retinal nerve fiber layer, ganglion cell layer or ganglion cell complex in any eye. Thus, we conclude from this exploratory research that the macular morphology differs between dyslexic and normal control subjects, as measured by OCT, especially in the parafovea at middle retinal segmentations.

Keywords: dyslexia; reading; retina; macula; fovea; parafovea; perifovea; optical coherence tomography; thickness; segmentation

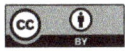

1. Introduction

Dyslexia has been defined as a neurodevelopmental disorder characterized by reading difficulties in the absence of psychiatric, neurological, auditory or visual disabilities [1]. This disorder has been estimated to affect between 5 and 15% of children and around 4% of adults in the general population [2].

The pathophysiology of dyslexia is still controversial and has been attributed to phonological, auditory or visual alterations [3,4]. A number of neuroimaging investigations focused on the central nervous system (CNS) have been performed so far to study normal [5] and abnormal reading process [2,6], and also reading interventions [7,8]. However, we have to keep in mind that the first steps of a successful reading process are entirely visual and are related to the retina, a part of the CNS located in the eye [9]. The retina is made up of a complex cell circuitry of neurons (photoreceptors, bipolar cells, horizontal cells, amacrine cells and ganglion cells) and glial cells (astrocytes, Müller cells and microglial cells) that are arranged into alternating layers of the nuclei and axons/synapses [9,10]. These layers can be individually segmented in vivo in cross-sectional scans, and their thickness quantified with a non-invasive and reproducible technology called optical coherence tomography (OCT), that achieves a high resolution in cross-sectional images (Figure 1a), similar to that obtained in histological sections [11]. OCT technology has been extensively used to study biomarkers in other CNS disorders [12,13].

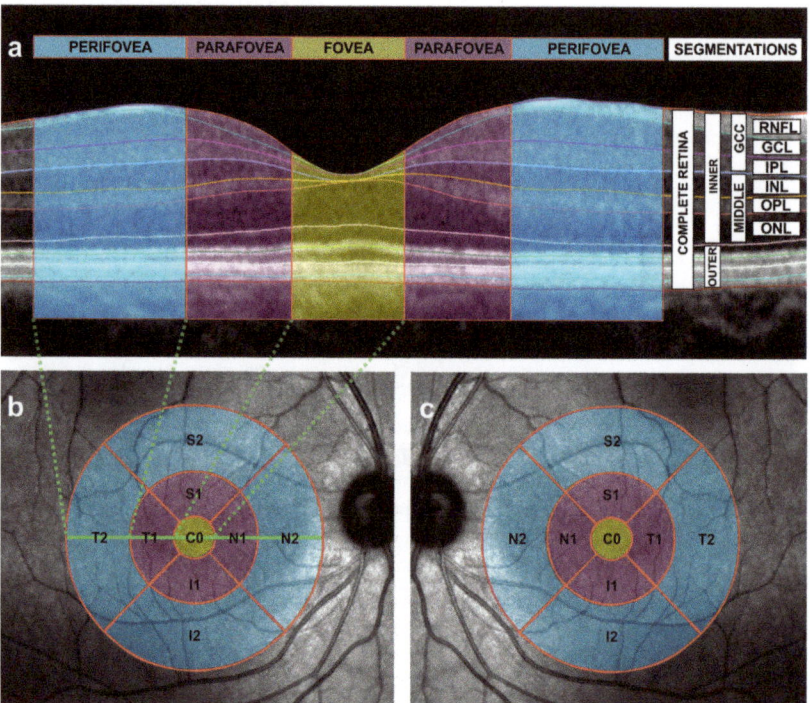

Figure 1. Cross-sectional and en face scans obtained by the means of optical coherence tomography (OCT). (**a**) Automatic segmentation of the different intraretinal layers in a cross-sectional OCT image of the macula from a right eye. The fovea is depicted in yellow, the parafoveal subfield in purple and the perifoveal subfield in blue. See Figure 1b,c for the corresponding en face representation of the fovea, parafovea and perifovea with the same color code as the one used in this figure. Dashed green lines indicate the limits of the temporal perifovea, the temporal parafovea and the fovea in relation to the en face image (see also Figure 1b). Segmentations are also shown. RNFL = retinal nerve fiber layer, GCL = ganglion cell layer (GCL), IPL= inner plexiform layer, INL = inner nuclear layer, OPL = outer plexiform layer, ONL = outer nuclear layer, GCC = ganglion cell complex, MIDDLE = middle retinal layers, INNER = inner retina, OUTER = outer retina. (**b**) Early Treatment Diabetic Retinopathy Study (ETDRS) grid with concentric circles of 1, 3 and 6 mm diameters of the right eye, showing nine sectors of the macula in an en face OCT image. The OCT device automatically estimates the mean thickness in microns for each sector and for each segmentation (see also Figure 1a). T = temporal, N = nasal, S = superior, I = inferior, C0 = fovea. Number 1 and number 2 refer to the inner

ring and the outer ring, respectively, and correspond to the parafovea (inner ring) and the perifovea (outer ring). The macula is depicted with the same color code as in Figure 1a (the fovea in yellow, the parafovea in purple and the perifovea in blue). The horizontal, solid, green line indicates the location of the cross-sectional scan of Figure 1a in the en face image. Dashed green lines indicate the limits of the temporal perifovea, the temporal parafovea and the fovea in relation to cross-sectional images (see Figure 1a). (c) Early Treatment Diabetic Retinopathy Study (ETDRS) grid with concentric circles of 1, 3 and 6 mm diameters of the left eye, showing nine sectors of the macula in an en face OCT image. The OCT device automatically estimates the mean thickness in microns for each sector and for each segmentation (see also Figure 1a). T = temporal, N = nasal, S = superior, I = inferior, C0 = fovea. Number 1 and number 2 refer to the inner ring and the outer ring, respectively, and correspond to the parafovea (inner ring) and the perifovea (outer ring). The macula is depicted with the same color code as in Figure 1a (the fovea in yellow, the parafovea in purple and the perifovea in blue).

Specifically, the reading process starts with the projection of a well-focused image of the text onto the central part of the retina, called the macula. Then, this macular image is encoded by photoreceptors in a process called phototransduction, and transmitted through the chain of neurons of the visual pathway to the brain cortex to be interpreted [14]. The macular region includes the fovea, the parafovea and the perifovea [10] (Figure 1a–c).

Despite the macula being such an important site for the reading process, no study is available about the macular morphology in dyslexia as far as we know. Thus, the aim of this research was to compare the thickness of different retinal segmentations between dyslexic subjects and normal controls at the macula, by the means of OCT.

2. Materials and Methods

2.1. Recruitment

In this study, dyslexic and normal controls were prospectively recruited from the patients attending the hospital for a routine ophthalmic review at the General University Reina Sofia Hospital of Murcia, Spain.

The inclusion criteria for the dyslexic group were: (1) Caucasian race; (2) Spanish as mother tongue; (3) aged under 25 years; (4) previous diagnosis of dyslexia confirmed by at least two different specialists; (5) refraction less than 6 spherical diopters and 2.5 cylinder diopters; (6) visual acuity of 20/25 or higher; (7) no history or findings of eye diseases or previous eye surgery; (8) no extraocular disease capable of modifying OCT measurements; (9) a reliable OCT scan (see below); (10) no other sensory, neurological, psychiatric, emotional or intellectual disorders; (11) no socio/economic significant disadvantage. Self-reported normal reader controls had the same inclusion criteria, except for criterion number 4. Only those participants not self-reporting reading difficulty and who correctly read aloud a simple 5-line paragraph text, without making a mistake or awkward pauses, were recruited in the control group.

2.2. Ophthalmic Examinations

All the patients underwent a complete ophthalmic examination in both eyes, including visual acuity, autorefraction, air pneumatic tonometry, biomicroscopy and funduscopy. If the candidates were eligible, they underwent posterior pole horizontal protocol with 768 A- and 61 B-scans taken 30 × 25 degrees centered at the fovea, using a Spectralis OCT spectral domain device with an eye-tracking system (software version 6.0; Heidelberg Engineering, Heidelberg, Germany).

The OCT examinations were performed in the morning, between 8:30 and 12:30 h, with pupil dilation. During this examination, the mean thickness of nine sectors was determined for each considered segmentation using the 1, 3, 6 mm diameter Early Treatment Diabetic Retinopathy Study protocol, that is one of the most used OCT en face patterns to study the macula, which considers the fovea, parafovea and perifovea subfields (Figure 1b,c). The position of the fovea was automatically determined by the device and checked by the same ophthalmologist (J.J.G.M.). Only reliable scans, with a signal strength over 20, were included. All the scans were performed by the same operator and inspected by the same experienced ophthalmologist (J.J.G.M.), in order to exclude eyes with segmentation errors, decentering or any other artifact. No manual corrections were made to the automatic segmentation performed by the prototype software. The examinations with decentrations, or with segmentation errors that could alter thickness estimation at any sector, were excluded.

Then, with a segmentation tool (Segmentation Technology; Heidelberg Engineering), the thickness values of the following segmentations were automatically obtained: complete retina, inner retina, outer retina, retinal nerve fiber layer (RNFL), ganglion cell layer (GCL), inner plexiform layer (IPL), inner nuclear layer (INL), outer plexiform layer (OPL), outer nuclear layer (ONL). The thickness value of the other segmentations was also obtained by summing up the thicknesses of the automatically obtained segmentations as follows: ganglion cell complex (RNFL + GCL + IPL), middle retina (INL + OPL + ONL), IPL + INL and OPL + ONL (Figure 1a). The thicknesses of OPL and ONL were not considered individually and were summed up, as was performed in previous works regarding autism [15] and glaucoma [16–18], because these two layers are hard to be conveniently separated in OCT images due to their similar reflectivity. A three-dimensional video (Video S1) has been made in order to better understand the integration of cross-sectional (Figure 1a) and en face OCT images (Figure 1b,c). Considering that neurons and glia in the human retina are organized in concentric rings around the fovea [19,20], we also summarized the thickness for all the mentioned segmentations considering the inner ring subfield ((S1 + N1 + I1 + T1)/4) and the outer ring subfield ((S2 + N2 + I2 + T2)/4) that correspond to the parafovea (purple ring in Figure 1b,c) and to the perifovea (blue ring in Figure 1b,c), respectively.

2.3. Statistical Analysis

The data analysis was conducted using SPSS version 22.0 (SPSS, Inc., Chicago, IL, USA). As there were no previous similar studies, no sample size calculation was performed in this investigation. The results of the right and left eyes were separately compared between the groups. Gender was compared between the groups by a Fisher's exact test. The quantitative variables were assessed for normality distribution by inspecting histograms and using the Shapiro–Wilk test. Normally distributed variables were expressed as the mean and standard deviation, while non-normally distributed values were expressed as the median and interquartile range. Comparisons between two normally distributed variables were performed with the unpaired Student's t-test. If at least one variable was non-normally distributed, the comparison between the groups was made by the Mann–Whitney test. A correction for multiple comparisons was not applied to this study in order to avoid the false-negative results [21]. A p-value less than 0.05 was considered statistically significant.

3. Results

The OCT examinations of one right eye from the dyslexic group and two left eyes from the control group were discarded due to segmentation errors at one or more sectors. Finally, 89 reliable OCT scans from 46 participants were selected in this study: 24 right eyes (7 men, 17 women) and 25 left eyes (8 men, 17 women) were selected from 25 normal controls. Moreover, 21 right eyes (7 men, 14 women) and 19 left eyes (5 men, 14 women) were included from 21 dyslexic subjects. The gender between the dyslexic and control groups did not differ when considering the right (p = 1, Fisher's exact test) or the left eyes (p = 0.749, Fisher's exact test).

Similarly, the mean age was not different between the groups for the right eyes (15.83 ± 3.81 years for dyslexics, with a range of 9 to 23 years, and 16.00 ± 4.11 for normal controls, with a range of 10 to 23 years, p = 0.889, unpaired Student's t-test) or for the left eyes (15.76 ± 3.75 years for dyslexics, with a range of 10 to 23 years, and 16.26 ± 3.97 for normal controls, with a range of 10 to 23 years, p = 0.672, unpaired Student's t-test).

The thicknesses in all four parafoveal sectors were significantly thicker in both the right and left eyes of the dyslexic group in the following segmentations: complete retina (Table S1), inner retina (Table S2), middle retina (INL + OPL + ONL) (Table S3) and OPL + ONL

(Table S4). Several macular sectors were also thicker in IPL (Table S5), INL (Table S6) and IPL + INL (Table S7) in dyslexia. Moreover, a foveal thickening was also observed in both eyes for OPL + ONL (and also for INL + ONL + OPL in the right eye) (Figure 2).

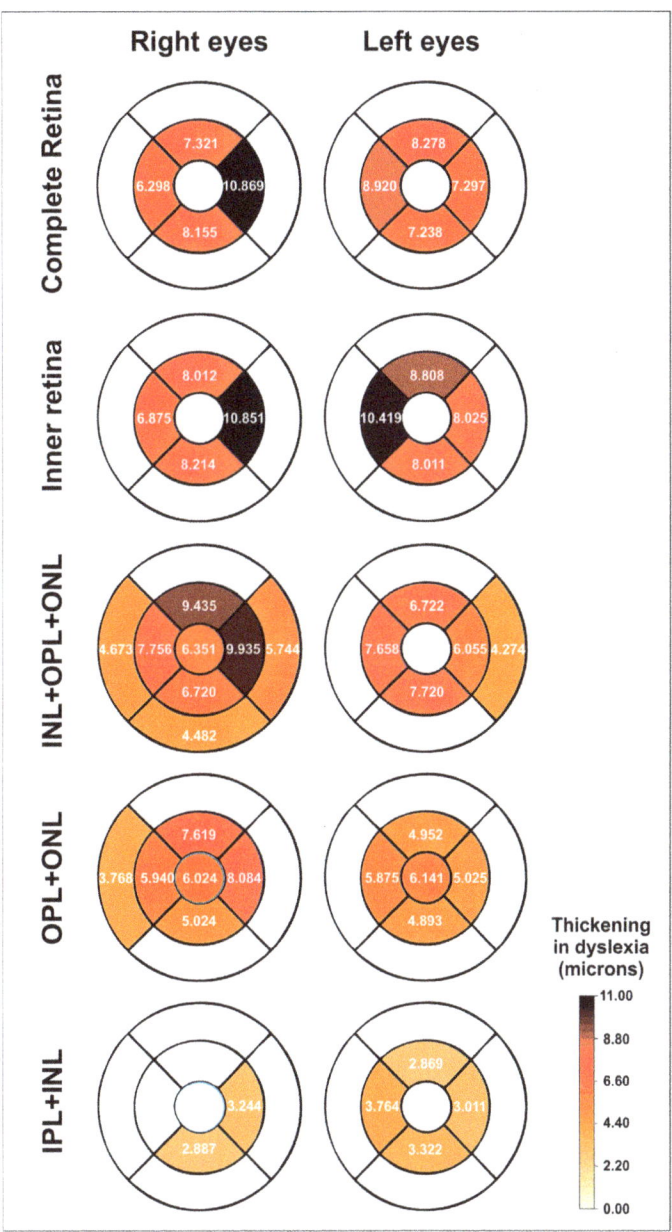

Figure 2. Schematic heatmaps of the statistically significant thickenings (expressed as microns) in the dyslexic group compared to the normal control group for the right and left eyes (mean differences in thickness) and for different segmentations. See also Figure 1a–c. White sectors indicate no significant differences. IPL = inner plexiform layer, INL = inner nuclear layer, OPL = outer plexiform layer, ONL = outer nuclear layer. See also Tables S1–S4 and S7.

In contrast, no thickness differences were observed between both the groups in any of the sectors of the retinal nerve fiber layer (RNFL) (Table S8), ganglion cell layer (GCL) (Table S9), ganglion cell complex (RNFL + GCL + IPL) (Table S10) or outer retina (Table S11) in either eye.

When considering the inner ring subfield (parafovea), we found that the complete retina, inner retina, middle retina (INL + OPL + ONL), OPL + ONL, IPL + INL and INL showed a higher thickness in the dyslexic group for both eyes, with IPL showing this difference only for the right eye (Table 1). The rest of the segmentations (outer retina, GCC, RNFL, GCL) did not present any significant differences in either eye (Table 1).

Table 1. Thickness comparison between the groups for the inner ring subfield (parafovea) in the ETDRS grid.

		Thickness of the Inner ETDRS Ring Subfield (Parafovea) Comparisons between Normal Controls and Dyslexic Subjects								
		Right Eyes (24 vs. 21)					Left Eyes (25 vs. 19)			
	Group	Mean	Std. Dev.	Mean Dif.	p (UTT)		Mean	Std. Dev.	Mean Dif.	p (UTT)
Complete retina	Control	330.63	10.25	−8.16	0.011		330.33	10.36	−7.93	0.019
	Dyslexia	338.79	10.32				338.26	11.04		
Inner retina	Control	251.08	8.72	−8.49	0.004		250.50	9.11	−8.82	0.006
	Dyslexia	259.57	10.07				259.32	10.98		
Outer retina	Control	79.48	2.12	0.30	0.599		79.87	2.46	0.94	0.176
	Dyslexia	79.18	1.60				78.93	1.89		
GCC	Control	114.38	5.52	0.58	0.777		113.29	4.60	−1.89	0.278
	Dyslexia	113.80	7.97				115.18	6.82		
INL + OPL + ONL	Control	137.31	6.73	−8.46	0.0002		137.38	6.51	−6.87	0.003
	Dyslexia	145.77	7.67				144.25	7.70		
ONNL	Control	98.19	5.73	−6.66	0.001		98.45	5.63	−5.18	0.010
	Dyslexia	104.85	6.94				103.63	7.07		
IPL + INL	Control	80.28	3.70	−2.55	0.036		80.14	3.86	−3.24	0.009
	Dyslexia	82.83	4.22				83.38	3.92		
RNFL	Control	21.01	2.59	0.99	0.142		20.24	1.33	0.17	0.681
	Dyslexia	20.02	1.66				20.07	1.45		
GCL	Control	52.21	2.71	0.34	0.758		51.84	2.67	−0.52	0.595
	Dyslexia	51.87	4.33				52.36	3.71		
IPL	Control	41.16	1.67	−0.74	0.310		41.21	1.76	−1.55	0.015
	Dyslexia	41.90	2.93				42.76	2.31		
INL	Control	39.13	2.61	−1.80	0.020		38.93	2.62	−1.69	0.025
	Dyslexia	40.93	2.34				40.62	2.05		

Right and left eyes were independently compared between the groups. The thickness results are expressed as microns. Statistically significant results are depicted in bold. Std. Dev = standard deviation, Dif. = difference, UTT = unpaired *t*-test, GCC = ganglion cell complex, RNFL = retinal nerve fiber layer, GCL = ganglion cell layer, IPL = inner plexiform layer, INL = inner nuclear layer, OPL = outer plexiform layer, ONL = outer nuclear layer.

In contrast, when dealing with the outer ring subfield (perifovea), only INL + OPL + ONL and INL showed a discrete increase of thickness in the dyslexia group, only when comparing the right eyes (Table 2).

Table 2. Thickness comparison between the groups for the outer ring subfield (perifovea) in the ETDRS grid.

		Thickness of the Outer ETDRS Ring Subfield (Perifovea) Comparisons between Normal Controls and Dyslexic Subjects							
		Right Eyes (24 vs. 21)				Left Eyes (25 vs. 19)			
	Group	Mean	Std. Dev.	Mean Dif.	p (UTT)	Mean	Std. Dev.	Mean Dif.	p (UTT)
Complete retina	Control	294.82	12.43	−4.66	0.256	294.38	10.64	−4.57	0.218
	Dyslexia	299.48	14.67			298.95	13.62		
Inner retina	Control	217.85	11.48	−4.35	0.271	217.14	9.97	−4.91	0.173
	Dyslexia	222.20	14.62			222.05	13.54		
Outer retina	Control	76.91	1.73	−0.42	0.380	77.20	1.67	0.29	0.564
	Dyslexia	77.33	1.46			76.91	1.62		
GCC	Control	100.31	6.96	−0.58	0.808	100.31	6.96	−0.58	0.804
	Dyslexia	100.89	8.60			100.89	8.60		
INL + OPL + ONL	Control	117.07	5.84	−4.58	**0.020**	117.30	5.81	−3.81	0.057
	Dyslexia	121.65	6.90			121.11	7.06		
ONP + ONL	Control	83.07	5.03	−3.31	0.051	83.27	4.97	−2.93	0.083
	Dyslexia	86.38	6.02			86.20	5.96		
IPL + INL	Control	63.64	3.42	−1.82	0.132	63.66	3.60	−1.71	0.165
	Dyslexia	65.46	4.55			65.37	4.41		
RNFL	Control	34.81	5.25	1.30	0.331	33.79	3.99	0.41	0.718
	Dyslexia	33.51	3.23			33.38	3.24		
GCL	Control	36.98	2.95	0.06	0.956	36.89	2.75	−0.16	0.871
	Dyslexia	36.92	4.38			37.05	3.87		
IPL	Control	29.64	1.97	−0.55	0.471	29.63	1.71	−0.83	0.258
	Dyslexia	30.19	2.97			30.46	2.75		
INL	Control	34.00	1.76	−1.27	**0.020**	34.03	2.23	−0.88	0.171
	Dyslexia	35.27	1.78			34.91	1.84		

Right and left eyes were independently compared between the groups. The thickness results are expressed as microns. Statistically significant results are depicted in bold. Std. Dev. = standard deviation, Dif. = difference, UTT = unpaired t-test, GCC = ganglion cell complex, RNFL = retinal nerve fiber layer, GCL = ganglion cell layer, IPL = inner plexiform layer, INL = inner nuclear layer, OPL = outer plexiform layer, ONL = outer nuclear layer.

4. Discussion

This study found parafoveal thickenings in both eyes of the dyslexic group for the middle retina, mainly the ONL-related segmentations, but also for the INL-related segmentations (Table 1). Remarkably, no difference was noted in the GCL-related segmentations or in the outer retina of right or left eyes. Furthermore, complete retina and inner retinal thickenings found at the parafovea in this study seem to be due to the middle retinal thickenings (Figure 1a; see also Table 1 and Tables S1–S4 and S7). Additionally, a foveal thickening was also observed in ONL + OPL (in both eyes) and INL + ONL + OPL (in the right eye).

The ONL contains photoreceptor cell bodies and the INL bipolar, amacrine and horizontal cells nuclei. OPL and IPL are made up of axons and synapses and connect the neighboring nuclear layers (ONL-INL and INL-GCL, respectively) [9]. In fact, the ONL and INL layers share a common embryological origin: the outer neuroblastic zone differentiates into ONL and INL after fetal week 10. Then, first synapses appear in the IPL and OPL by fetal week 12 [10]. ONL and INL the somata are displaced during normal foveal development (from fetal week 22 to postpartum month 45): photoreceptor cell bodies (ONL) present a centripetal displacement toward the foveal center with cellular packing and elongation, while INL and GCL have centrifugal displacement to the foveal rim [10]. One possible explanation for the thickenings found in this study is a disorder in foveal development due to a gap between these two movements in the opposite direction. In this way, orientation of the somata and the axons of ONL- and INL-related cells could result in more vertical increasing of the thickness of these layers. This mechanism has been proposed to explain some similar retinal features found in the eyes of preterm patients with foveal immaturity [22]. Other alternative explanations for the found thickenings could be a neuronal/glial population increase, cell size augmentation or an extracellular expansion in the affected segmentations. More studies are warranted to elucidate this question.

A genetically determined disorder in foveal development could bring about the findings of the present study. This hypothesis is consistent with the fact that dyslexia presents a high degree of heritability (70% or even more), whereas the environment has little effect [23–25].

As a matter of fact, some genetic polymorphisms have been detected to be much more prevalent in dyslexia. These polymorphisms are in relation to abnormal axonal growth and defective neural migration [26–28], and have been associated with alterations in the development of cortico-cortical and cortico-thalamic circuits in dyslexia [2,29], so they may similarly lead to the retinal differences detected in this study.

The highest thickenings found in this study were located at the parafovea, although alterations at the fovea, and even at some perifoveal sectors, were also present in OPL + ONL and INL + OPL + ONL segmentations (Figure 2). The fovea captures the visual field one degree around the fixation point, while the parafovea is surrounding the fovea up to five degrees from the fixation point [30,31].

The fovea and the parafovea work together in the reading process, because, although the fovea is oriented to the target word, the parafovea previews the next words to facilitate further foveal processing [32,33]. In fact, parafoveal recognition of embedded letters and words has been proven to be worse in dyslexic subjects than in normal controls [34–36]. Furthermore, reduced and delayed parafoveal preview benefits have been associated with dyslexia [37–40].

Thus, the thickenings found in this study could constitute the morphological correlation of parafoveal dysfunction in dyslexia. These thickenings may theoretically cause a higher level of light scattering transmitted to the outer segments of photoreceptors, where the phototransduction takes place, and potentially a subsequent loss of sensitivity [10]. The other possibility is that the found thickenings could be related to a change in the arrangement of the photoreceptors and/or Müller cells, as suggested above. An incorrect arrangement of these cells may induce an incorrect angle of incidence of light and a subsequent reduction of sensitivity due to the Stiles–Crawford effect of the first kind [41,42]. These, or other causes associated to these thickenings, may alter parafoveal preview function. Further study is required in this sense.

It is also remarkable that the thickening in all four parafoveal sectors (360 degrees) found herein is consistent with the fact that dyslexia is present in all languages, independently of the reading direction going from left to right (English, Spanish, French, German), from right to left (Hebrew or Arabic) or from top to bottom (Japanese, Chinese) [6].

This exploratory research also has its limitations. First, the sample size is small and the outcomes should be studied in larger groups, but we found significant results. Moreover, the facts that the comparisons have been calculated separately for the right and the left eyes and that the found differences are so similar in both eyes, affecting the same segmentations and with analogous disparities, reinforce the validity of our results (Figure 2). Second, the participants included in this study are mainly adolescents and young adults, so we cannot extrapolate our results to other age groups. Third, this study is cross-sectional, so we cannot know whether the found differences are stable over time and whether reading interventions are able to remodel retinal structures, similarly to what has been found in other investigations on the CNS in dyslexia [7,8]. Fourth, the grouping of this study is based on a diagnosis and not on specific reading measurements. Using a categorical method to create the groups does not permit to explore a quantitative correlation between reading measurements (for example, reading speed) and OCT parameters. However, we have to keep in mind that this is an exploratory investigation. Further works should deal with these relationships. Fifth, it should be pointed out that the nomenclature of the inner and outer retina, as defined by the OCT device used in this study (Spectralis, Heidelberg Engineering), is inexact (Figure 1). The inner and outer retina are major divisions in both neurobiology and vascular biology. The outer retina includes the OPL, ONL, photoreceptors and retinal pigment epithelium, and receives blood supply from choroidal circulation, whereas the inner retinal layers are dependent on retinal circulation [43]. However, this fact does not affect the results of this study. Sixth, this study is limited in analyzing morphological results. Further functional studies (i.e., mERG) in relation to morphological differences should be investigated in further studies. Seventh, the OCT examinations were only analyzed by one expert, so inter-variability agreement cannot be assessed. However, all the examinations fulfilled the reliability criteria. Finally, this study is limited to describe morphological differences in the macula of dyslexic subjects, so we cannot determine if these findings are causes or consequences, or the parallel manifestations in the pathophysiology of dyslexia: if these morphological findings were the cause, dyslexia could be primarily a retinal disorder, as suggested above. If they were the consequence or a parallel manifestation, dyslexia would be capable of remodeling retinal structures, as is done in other CNS structures [2,6,44]. Thus, the macula could be a privileged and accessible site to study dyslexia by using a fast, inexpensive and non-invasive technique, such as OCT. Further studies are required in this sense. Nevertheless, our significant results open a new horizon for the investigation of dyslexia.

5. Conclusions

From this exploratory research, we conclude that the macular morphology differs in dyslexic and normal controls, especially in the parafovea.

Supplementary Materials: The following supporting information can be downloaded at: https://www.mdpi.com/article/10.3390/jcm12062356/s1, Video S1 and Tables S1–S11 have been added as supplementary material. Video S1. Three-dimensional (3D) video that dynamically combines the cross-sectional and the en face OCT scans of the macula from a right eye. The cross-sectional scans that configure the 3D surface of the macula progressively disappear, while the two-dimensional image of the en face scan remains. See also Figure 1a,b.

Author Contributions: Conceptualization, J.J.G.-M.; Methodology, J.J.G.-M., P.S.-C., C.G.-M., M.D.-P.-M., V.Z.-M., M.D.P.-D. and M.D.-R.-V.; Formal analysis, J.J.G.-M., N.B.-M., C.G.-M., E.R.-V., M.D.-P.-M., V.Z.-M., M.D.P.-D. and M.D.-R.-V.; Investigation, P.S.-C., C.G.-M., E.R.-V., M.D.P.-D. and M.D.-R.-V.; Data curation, J.J.G.-M., N.B.-M. and P.S.-C.; Writing—original draft, J.J.G.-M., N.B.-M., P.S.-C., C.G.-M., E.R.-V., M.D.-P.-M., V.Z.-M., M.D.P.-D. and M.D.-R.-V.; Writing—review & editing, J.J.G.-M., N.B.-M., P.S.-C., C.G.-M., E.R.-V., M.D.-P.-M., V.Z.-M., M.D.P.-D. and M.D.-R.-V.; Supervision, J.J.G.-M. and M.D.-R.-V. All authors have read and agreed to the published version of the manuscript.

Funding: This research received no external funding.

Institutional Review Board Statement: The study was approved by the Local Ethics Committee at the University General Reina Sofia Hospital of Murcia, Spain (protocol 005/2017), and adhered to the Declaration of Helsinki criteria.

Informed Consent Statement: The participants or their legal representative signed an informed consent form.

Data Availability Statement: The data sets generated and/or analyzed during this study are available from the corresponding author on reasonable request.

Acknowledgments: This work has been done in part with the collaboration of members assigned to the research team of Murcia and Valencia, pertaining to the ophthalmology network OFTARED (RD16-0008), as well as the members of the inflammatory diseases network RICORS (RD21/0002/0032) of the Institute of Health Carlos III (ISCIII), Spanish Government (Madrid, Spain). We would like to thank Jose Manuel Tamarit (Heidelberg Engineering, Heidelberg, Germany) for his technical help with the OCT device and Guadalupe Ruiz (Statistics Department, FFIS-IMIB, Murcia, Spain) for her statistical assistance in the data analysis of this study. The preliminary results of this study were presented during the Association for Research in Vision and Ophthalmology (ARVO) Annual Meeting, originally scheduled for 2–6 May in San Francisco, CA, USA, 2021, but finally presented in a

Virtual Meeting. The final results of this study were presented at the 23rd Congress of the European Association for Vision and Eye Research (EVER), 13–15 October 2022 in Valencia, Spain.

Conflicts of Interest: The authors have no relevant financial or non-financial interests to disclose.

References

1. American Psychiatric Association (Ed.) *Diagnostic and Statistical Manual of Mental Disorders: DSM-5*, 5th ed.; American Psychiatric Association: Washington, DC, USA, 2013; ISBN 9780890425541.
2. Soriano-Ferrer, M.; Piedra Martínez, E. A Review of the Neurobiological Basis of Dyslexia in the Adult Population. *Neurologia* **2017**, *32*, 50–57. [CrossRef] [PubMed]
3. Stein, J. What Is Developmental Dyslexia? *Brain Sci.* **2018**, *8*, E26. [CrossRef] [PubMed]
4. Werth, R. Is Developmental Dyslexia Due to a Visual and Not a Phonological Impairment? *Brain Sci.* **2021**, *11*, 1313. [CrossRef]
5. Wandell, B.A.; Le, R.K. Diagnosing the Neural Circuitry of Reading. *Neuron* **2017**, *96*, 298–311. [CrossRef]
6. Shaywitz, S.E.; Shaywitz, J.E.; Shaywitz, B.A. Dyslexia in the 21st Century. *Curr. Opin. Psychiatry* **2021**, *34*, 80–86. [CrossRef]
7. Perdue, M.V.; Mahaffy, K.; Vlahcevic, K.; Wolfman, E.; Erbeli, F.; Richlan, F.; Landi, N. Reading Intervention and Neuroplasticity: A Systematic Review and Meta-Analysis of Brain Changes Associated with Reading Intervention. *Neurosci. Biobehav.* **2022**, *132*, 465–494. [CrossRef]
8. Braid, J.; Richlan, F. The Functional Neuroanatomy of Reading Intervention. *Front. Neurosci.* **2022**, *16*, 921931. [CrossRef] [PubMed]
9. Purves, D.; Augustine, G.J.; Fitzpatrick, D.; Hall, W.C.; LaMantia, A.-S.; Mooney, R.D.; Platt, M.L.; White, L.E. (Eds.) *Neuroscience*, 6th ed.; Oxford University Press: New York, NY, USA, 2018; ISBN 9781605353807.
10. Bringmann, A.; Wiedemann, P. *The Fovea: Structure, Function, Development, and Tractional Disorders*, 1st ed.; Elsevier: Waltham, MA, USA, 2021; ISBN 9780323904674.
11. Vajzovic, L.; Hendrickson, A.E.; O'Connell, R.V.; Clark, L.A.; Tran-Viet, D.; Possin, D.; Chiu, S.J.; Farsiu, S.; Toth, C.A. Maturation of the Human Fovea: Correlation of Spectral-Domain Optical Coherence Tomography Findings with Histology. *Am. J. Ophthalmol.* **2012**, *154*, 779–789.e2. [CrossRef]
12. Vujosevic, S.; Parra, M.M.; Hartnett, M.E.; O'Toole, L.; Nuzzi, A.; Limoli, C.; Villani, E.; Nucci, P. Optical Coherence Tomography as Retinal Imaging Biomarker of Neuroinflammation/Neurodegeneration in Systemic Disorders in Adults and Children. *Eye* **2023**, *37*, 203–219. [CrossRef]
13. Xie, J.S.; Donaldson, L.; Margolin, E. The Use of Optical Coherence Tomography in Neurology: A Review. *Brain* **2022**, *145*, 4160–4177. [CrossRef] [PubMed]
14. Beauchamp, G.R.; Kosmorsky, G.S. The Neurophysiology of Reading. *Int. Ophthalmol. Clin.* **1989**, *29*, 16–19. [CrossRef]
15. Garcia-Medina, J.J.; del-Rio-Vellosillo, M.; Palazón-Cabanes, A.; Tudela-Molino, M.; Gómez-Molina, C.; Guardiola-Fernández, A.; Villegas-Pérez, M.P. Mapping the thickness changes on retinal layers segmented by spectral-domain optical coherence tomography using the posterior pole program in glaucoma. *Arch. Soc. Esp. Oftalmol.* **2018**, *93*, 263–273. [CrossRef]
16. Garcia-Medina, J.J.; Del-Rio-Vellosillo, M.; Palazon-Cabanes, A.; Pinazo-Duran, M.D.; Zanon-Moreno, V.; Villegas-Perez, M.P. Glaucomatous Maculopathy: Thickness Differences on Inner and Outer Macular Layers between Ocular Hypertension and Early Primary Open-Angle Glaucoma Using 8 × 8 Posterior Pole Algorithm of SD-OCT. *J. Clin. Med.* **2020**, *9*, E1503. [CrossRef] [PubMed]
17. Garcia-Medina, J.J.; Rotolo, M.; Rubio-Velazquez, E.; Pinazo-Duran, M.D.; Del-Rio-Vellosillo, M. Macular Structure-Function Relationships of All Retinal Layers in Primary Open-Angle Glaucoma Assessed by Microperimetry and 8 × 8 Posterior Pole Analysis of OCT. *J. Clin. Med.* **2021**, *10*, 5009. [CrossRef] [PubMed]
18. Garcia-Medina, J.J.; García-Piñero, M.; Del-Río-Vellosillo, M.; Fares-Valdivia, J.; Ragel-Hernández, A.B.; Martínez-Saura, S.; Cárcel-López, M.D.; Zanon-Moreno, V.; Pinazo-Duran, M.D.; Villegas-Pérez, M.P. Comparison of Foveal, Macular, and Peripapillary Intraretinal Thicknesses Between Autism Spectrum Disorder and Neurotypical Subjects. *Investig. Ophthalmol. Vis. Sci.* **2017**, *58*, 5819–5826. [CrossRef] [PubMed]
19. Curcio, C.A.; Sloan, K.R.; Kalina, R.E.; Hendrickson, A.E. Human Photoreceptor Topography. *J. Comp. Neurol.* **1990**, *292*, 497–523. [CrossRef]
20. Hussey, K.A.; Hadyniak, S.E.; Johnston, R.J. Patterning and Development of Photoreceptors in the Human Retina. *Front. Cell Dev. Biol.* **2022**, *10*, 878350. [CrossRef]
21. Rothman, K.J. No Adjustments Are Needed for Multiple Comparisons. *Epidemiology* **1990**, *1*, 43–46. [CrossRef]
22. Sjöstrand, J.; Rosén, R.; Nilsson, M.; Popovic, Z. Arrested Foveal Development in Preterm Eyes: Thickening of the Outer Nuclear Layer and Structural Redistribution Within the Fovea. *Investig. Ophthalmol. Vis. Sci.* **2017**, *58*, 4948. [CrossRef]
23. Kirkpatrick, R.M.; Legrand, L.N.; Iacono, W.G.; McGue, M. A Twin and Adoption Study of Reading Achievement: Exploration of Shared-Environmental and Gene-Environment-Interaction Effects. *Learn. Individ. Differ.* **2011**, *21*, 368–375. [CrossRef]
24. Astrom, R.L.; Wadsworth, S.J.; Olson, R.K.; Willcutt, E.G.; DeFries, J.C. Genetic and Environmental Etiologies of Reading Difficulties: DeFries–Fulker Analysis of Reading Performance Data from Twin Pairs and Their Non-Twin Siblings. *Learn. Individ. Differ.* **2012**, *22*, 365–369. [CrossRef] [PubMed]

25. Erbeli, F.; Rice, M.; Paracchini, S. Insights into Dyslexia Genetics Research from the Last Two Decades. *Brain Sci.* **2021**, *12*, 27. [CrossRef] [PubMed]
26. Massinen, S.; Hokkanen, M.-E.; Matsson, H.; Tammimies, K.; Tapia-Páez, I.; Dahlström-Heuser, V.; Kuja-Panula, J.; Burghoorn, J.; Jeppsson, K.E.; Swoboda, P.; et al. Increased Expression of the Dyslexia Candidate Gene DCDC2 Affects Length and Signaling of Primary Cilia in Neurons. *PLoS ONE* **2011**, *6*, e20580. [CrossRef]
27. Tarkar, A.; Loges, N.T.; Slagle, C.E.; Francis, R.; Dougherty, G.W.; Tamayo, J.V.; Shook, B.; Cantino, M.; Schwartz, D.; Jahnke, C.; et al. DYX1C1 Is Required for Axonemal Dynein Assembly and Ciliary Motility. *Nat. Genet.* **2013**, *45*, 995–1003. [CrossRef] [PubMed]
28. Diaz, R.; Kronenberg, N.M.; Martinelli, A.; Liehm, P.; Riches, A.C.; Gather, M.C.; Paracchini, S. KIAA0319 Influences Cilia Length, Cell Migration and Mechanical Cell-Substrate Interaction. *Sci. Rep.* **2022**, *12*, 722. [CrossRef] [PubMed]
29. Thomas, T.; Khalaf, S.; Grigorenko, E.L. A Systematic Review and Meta-Analysis of Imaging Genetics Studies of Specific Reading Disorder. *Cogn. Neuropsychol.* **2021**, *38*, 179–204. [CrossRef]
30. Larson, A.M.; Loschky, L.C. The Contributions of Central versus Peripheral Vision to Scene Gist Recognition. *J. Vis.* **2009**, *9*, 6. [CrossRef] [PubMed]
31. Loschky, L.C.; Szaffarczyk, S.; Beugnet, C.; Young, M.E.; Boucart, M. The Contributions of Central and Peripheral Vision to Scene-Gist Recognition with a 180° Visual Field. *J. Vis.* **2019**, *19*, 15. [CrossRef] [PubMed]
32. Schotter, E.R.; Angele, B.; Rayner, K. Parafoveal Processing in Reading. *Atten. Percept. Psychophys.* **2012**, *74*, 5–35. [CrossRef]
33. Pan, Y.; Frisson, S.; Jensen, O. Neural Evidence for Lexical Parafoveal Processing. *Nat. Commun.* **2021**, *12*, 5234. [CrossRef]
34. Bouma, H.; Legein, C.P. Foveal and Parafoveal Recognition of Letters and Words by Dyslexics and by Average Readers. *Neuropsychologia* **1977**, *15*, 69–80. [CrossRef]
35. Geiger, G.; Lettvin, J.Y. Peripheral Vision in Persons with Dyslexia. *N. Engl. J. Med.* **1987**, *316*, 1238–1243. [CrossRef]
36. Geiger, G.; Cattaneo, C.; Galli, R.; Pozzoli, U.; Lorusso, M.L.; Facoetti, A.; Molteni, M. Wide and Diffuse Perceptual Modes Characterize Dyslexics in Vision and Audition. *Perception* **2008**, *37*, 1745–1764. [CrossRef] [PubMed]
37. Jones, M.W.; Ashby, J.; Branigan, H.P. Dyslexia and Fluency: Parafoveal and Foveal Influences on Rapid Automatized Naming. *J. Exp. Psychol. Hum. Percept. Perform.* **2013**, *39*, 554–567. [CrossRef] [PubMed]
38. Yan, M.; Pan, J.; Laubrock, J.; Kliegl, R.; Shu, H. Parafoveal Processing Efficiency in Rapid Automatized Naming: A Comparison between Chinese Normal and Dyslexic Children. *J. Exp. Child Psychol.* **2013**, *115*, 579–589. [CrossRef] [PubMed]
39. Silva, S.; Faísca, L.; Araújo, S.; Casaca, L.; Carvalho, L.; Petersson, K.M.; Reis, A. Too Little or Too Much? Parafoveal Preview Benefits and Parafoveal Load Costs in Dyslexic Adults. *Ann. Dyslexia* **2016**, *66*, 187–201. [CrossRef]
40. Kirkby, J.A.; Barrington, R.S.; Drieghe, D.; Liversedge, S.P. Parafoveal Processing and Transposed-Letter Effects in Dyslexic Reading. *Dyslexia* **2022**, *28*, 359–374. [CrossRef]
41. Morris, H.J.; Blanco, L.; Codona, J.L.; Li, S.L.; Choi, S.S.; Doble, N. Directionality of Individual Cone Photoreceptors in the Parafoveal Region. *Vis. Res.* **2015**, *117*, 67–80. [CrossRef]
42. Tschulakow, A.V.; Oltrup, T.; Bende, T.; Schmelzle, S.; Schraermeyer, U. The Anatomy of the Foveola Reinvestigated. *PeerJ* **2018**, *6*, e4482. [CrossRef]
43. Campbell, J.P.; Zhang, M.; Hwang, T.S.; Bailey, S.T.; Wilson, D.J.; Jia, Y.; Huang, D. Detailed Vascular Anatomy of the Human Retina by Projection-Resolved Optical Coherence Tomography Angiography. *Sci. Rep.* **2017**, *7*, 42201. [CrossRef]
44. Kim, S.K. Recent Update on Reading Disability (Dyslexia) Focused on Neurobiology. *Clin. Exp. Pediatr.* **2021**, *64*, 497–503. [CrossRef] [PubMed]

Disclaimer/Publisher's Note: The statements, opinions and data contained in all publications are solely those of the individual author(s) and contributor(s) and not of MDPI and/or the editor(s). MDPI and/or the editor(s) disclaim responsibility for any injury to people or property resulting from any ideas, methods, instructions or products referred to in the content.

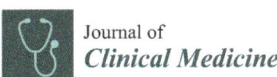

Article

Discriminating Healthy Optic Discs and Visible Optic Disc Drusen on Fundus Autofluorescence and Color Fundus Photography Using Deep Learning—A Pilot Study

Raphael Diener *, Jost Lennart Lauermann, Nicole Eter and Maximilian Treder

Department of Ophthalmology, University of Muenster Medical Center, 48149 Muenster, Germany
* Correspondence: raphael.diener@ukmuenster.de; Tel.: +49-251-835-6001

Abstract: The aim of this study was to use deep learning based on a deep convolutional neural network (DCNN) for automated image classification of healthy optic discs (OD) and visible optic disc drusen (ODD) on fundus autofluorescence (FAF) and color fundus photography (CFP). In this study, a total of 400 FAF and CFP images of patients with ODD and healthy controls were used. A pre-trained multi-layer Deep Convolutional Neural Network (DCNN) was trained and validated independently on FAF and CFP images. Training and validation accuracy and cross-entropy were recorded. Both generated DCNN classifiers were tested with 40 FAF and CFP images (20 ODD and 20 controls). After the repetition of 1000 training cycles, the training accuracy was 100%, the validation accuracy was 92% (CFP) and 96% (FAF), respectively. The cross-entropy was 0.04 (CFP) and 0.15 (FAF). The sensitivity, specificity, and accuracy of the DCNN for classification of FAF images was 100%. For the DCNN used to identify ODD on color fundus photographs, sensitivity was 85%, specificity 100%, and accuracy 92.5%. Differentiation between healthy controls and ODD on CFP and FAF images was possible with high specificity and sensitivity using a deep learning approach.

Keywords: deep learning; artificial intelligence; optic disc drusen; visible optic disc drusen; optic disc drusen; deep convolutional neural network; DCNN; inceptionv3

1. Introduction

Optic disc drusen (ODD) are acellular deposits that are located in the optic nerve head of 0.3% to 2.0% of the population [1,2].

In children and younger individuals, ODD are mostly buried deep in the optic nerve head [3,4]. They can be diagnosed using various imaging techniques, such as B-scan ultrasonography or, more recently, swept source (SS) or enhanced depth imaging (EDI) optical coherence tomography (OCT) [5,6]. Most of these cases are asymptomatic [7].

Due to an increase in drusen number, drusen growth or age-related thinning of the overlying retinal nerve fiber layer, ODD become visible with age and can, therefore, be detected on color fundus photography (CFP), fundus autofluorescence (FAF), and ophthalmoscopy [7]. Visible ODD are associated with visual field defects in up to 87% of cases [2,8–10]. Consequently, they are associated with high clinical relevance for visual function [11].

Because of the widespread use of multimodal imaging technologies as well as the digital fundus cameras for eye screening programs, there is an increasing amount of data to be analyzed by ophthalmologists, and therefore, a remarkable interest in the automated screening for optic nerve pathologies, such as ODD.

Artificial intelligence using deep learning (DL), a subtype of machine learning (ML), is used to solve complex and large-scale problems, such as speech and image recognition and language processing. The three most popular DL models are recurrent neural networks (RNNs), generative adversarial networks (GANs), and convolution neural networks (CNNs), which are particularly well suited for different tasks depending on their architecture.

RNNs are widely used in natural language processing and speech recognition tasks, where the input data are sequential in nature, such as text or speech. They use feedback connections that allow previous outputs to be used as inputs for subsequent processing, enabling the network to persist information across multiple steps and analyze complex dependencies in the data [12].

GANs have been applied to generative modeling tasks, such as image generation. They consist of two parts, a generator and a discriminator, that compete with each other to generate new data samples that are indistinguishable from real data [12].

CNNs are designed specifically for image classification tasks and are particularly well suited for recognizing patterns and features in images and have revolutionized data processing in medicine, especially in image-centric disciplines [12], such as Dermatology [13], Radiology [14], Pathology [15], and Ophthalmology [12,16]. In this context, CNNs have already been successfully used for automated image analysis using color fundus images for a number of ophthalmologic diseases with high prevalence, including glaucoma [17], diabetic retinopathy [18], and age-related macular degeneration [19].

ML and DL algorithms have several inherent limitations, including the need for very large, accurate datasets for learning. To overcome this limitation, transfer learning, which uses an already pre-trained deep learning algorithm can be used [19–21].

The aim of this study was to evaluate the use of a pre-trained CNN for the automated classification of visible ODD and healthy optic discs on fundus autofluorescence (FAF) and color fundus photography (CFP).

2. Materials and Methods

This study adhered to the tenets of the Declaration of Helsinki. Informed consent was waived due to the retrospective nature of the study and the fully anonymized usage of the database.

2.1. Patient and Image Selection

Patients with a clinical diagnosis of ODD and color fundus photography and fundus autofluorescence image of the optic disc were included in this study. Patients with no evidence of an optic disc pathology as determined by an ophthalmologist were defined as controls.

Images were chosen from a database of the Eye Clinics of Muenster University Hospital, compiled between January 2015 and January 2020. A total of 480 CFP and FAF images of the ODD and control group were used. All images were focused on the optic nerve head and were obtained using the same fundus autofluorescence (Spectralis, Heidelberg Engineering, Heidelberg, Germany) and color fundus photography (Visucam 500, Carl Zeiss Meditec AG, Jena, Germany) device. FAF devices produce greyscale images, whereas CFP devices produce Red-Green-Blue (RGB) images.

Inclusion criteria were selected in which drusen were visible in FAF as hyperfluorescent material. Images with buried optic disc drusen that were only visible in sonography or OCT were excluded.

All images were saved as JPEG files and had an input size of $299 \times 299 \times 3$ pixels.

2.2. Deep Learning

Training and validation of the DL model (InceptionV3) were performed using TensorFlow™ (Google Inc., Mountain View, CA, USA), which is an open-source software program developed by Google. It provides a high-level interface for designing and training DL models [20,22–25]. InceptionV3 is a DCNN designed for image classification tasks that was introduced by Szegedy et al. in 2015 [22]. It uses a modular architecture with multiple parallel convolutional paths and a concatenation layer that merges the result. This allows the network to capture both global and local features in the input image. Each layer takes an input and produces an output, which becomes an input to the next processing layer, creating a deep architecture. In each successive layer, the data were represented in an increasingly more abstract way. All layers, with the exception of the last layer, were pre-trained with an ImageNet [26] data set consisting of more than 14 million images of different objects and scenes. InceptionV3 can be fine-tuned for specific image-classification tasks with smaller datasets, which allows for faster and more accurate results. For this study, the last layer was trained with our ophthalmic dataset [27,28].

Two deep learning models were independently trained and validated using 120 FAF photos (ODD: $n = 60$; healthy: $n = 60$) and 120 CFP images (ODD: $n = 60$; healthy: $n = 60$) over the course of 1000 training steps (Figure 1). The training and validation accuracy, as well as the cross-entropy, were calculated in each of the training steps to evaluate the effectiveness of both training strategies. Forty FAF and 40 CFP photos (OOD: $n = 20$, healthy: $n = 20$) were used to assess the performance of both the developed DCNN models once the pre-training was completed (FAF and CFP). The 40 FAF and 40 CFP images used for testing were excluded from the dataset before training and validation of the algorithm were performed. The algorithm, therefore, had no access to the test data set during training and validation. Accordingly, the performance of the algorithm could be tested without bias.

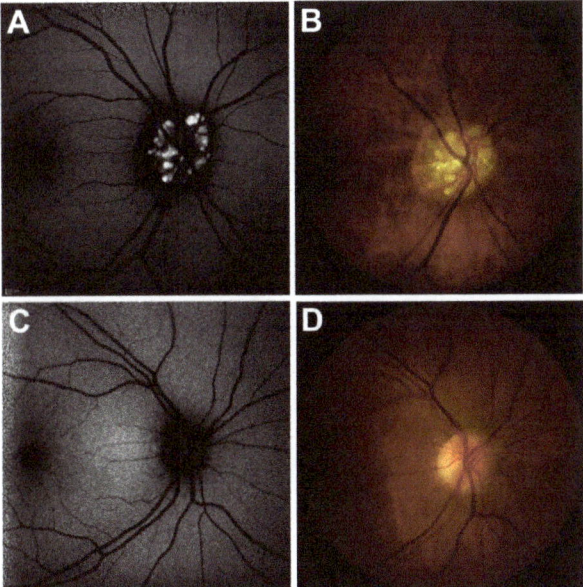

Figure 1. Fundus autofluorescence (**A,C**) and color fundus photography images (**B,D**) were used independently for training of the two different classifiers.

2.3. Statistics

SPSS was used to perform the statistics (IBM SPSS Statistics 23.0; IBM, Armonk, NY, USA). For descriptive statistics, Prism was utilized (Prism 7, GraphPad Software, Inc. San Diego, CA, USA). Data administration was carried out using Microsoft Excel (Microsoft® Excel® for Mac 2011, 14.6.2; Microsoft®, Redmond, WA, USA).

Mean differences in the probability scores of the two classifiers were verified with Mann–Whitney U-test for independent samples. The level of significance was defined as $p < 0.05$.

Using a 2 × 2 table, the sensitivity, specificity, and accuracy were computed. Both the DL procedure and the testing were repeated with the same data set to enable the evaluation of the precision of the repeatability of the ODD testing score. Coefficients of variation were computed to evaluate the precision. Bland–Altman plots were employed to evaluate repeatability.

3. Results

3.1. Performance of the Training Process

Both classifiers for FAF and CFP images had a training accuracy of 100% after 1000 performed training steps. The validation accuracy of the classifier for CFP and FAF images was 92% and 96%, respectively. There were no notable differences in the course of the curves of the training and the validation accuracy. The cross-entropy of both classifiers constantly decreased and was 0.15 (CFP images) and 0.04 (FAF images) after completion of the training process, as seen in Figure 2.

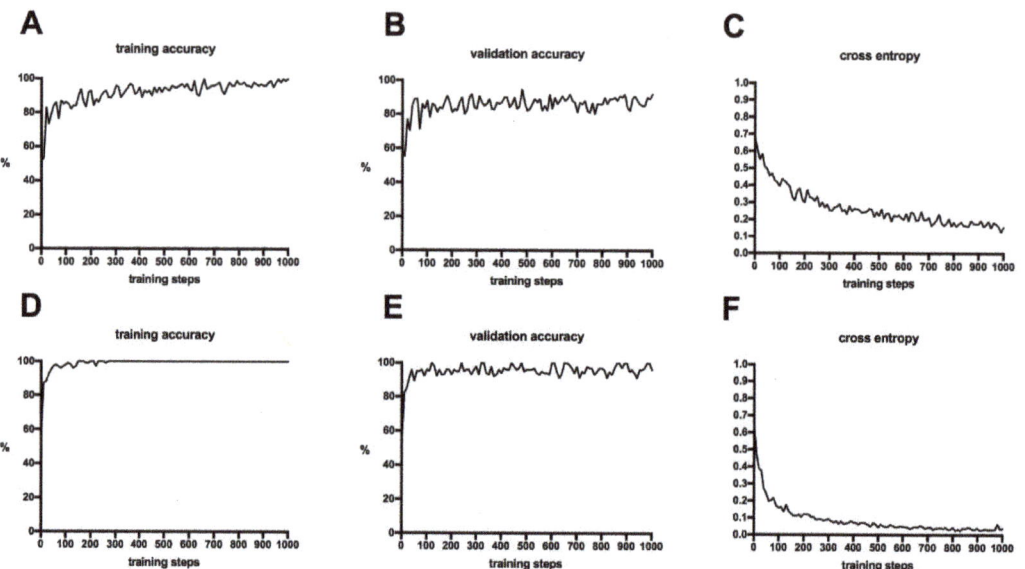

Figure 2. The graphs show the development of the training accuracy, validation accuracy, and cross-entropy of the two classifiers trained with color fundus photography (**A–C**) and fundus autofluorescence (**D–F**).

3.2. Testing of the Classifiers

All FAF images of both ODD and healthy test patients were correctly diagnosed by the classifier trained on this image modality. Consequently, sensitivity, specificity, and accuracy of this classifier were 100%, as shown in Table 1. The mean ODD testing scores for the ODD testing group's photos were 0.91 ± 0.15, and 0.05 ± 0.07 for the healthy control group's images. The mean healthy testing scores for the ODD testing group's images were 0.09 ± 0.15, and for the healthy control group's images, they were 0.95 ± 0.07.

Table 1. All fundus autofluorescence images of patients with ODD and normal optic discs were correctly identified, therefore, the sensitivity and specificity of the classifier were 100%.

	ODD Testing Group	Healthy Testing Group
Positive	n = 20	n = 0
Negative	n = 0	n = 20

ODD = Optic Disc Drusen.

All CFP images of the healthy test group were correctly diagnosed by the classifier whose last layer was trained with 120 CFP images. Three CFP images of patients with ODD were misdiagnosed by this classifier. Therefore, this classifier had a sensitivity of 85%, a specificity of 100% and an accuracy of 92.5%, as shown in Table 2.

Table 2. All color fundus photography images from healthy patients were correctly identified, whereas 3 CFP images from patients with ODD were misdiagnosed. Therefore, the sensitivity was 85%, and specificity was 100%.

	ODD Testing Group	Healthy Testing Group
Positive	$n = 17$	$n = 0$
Negative	$n = 3$	$n = 20$

ODD = Optic Disc Drusen.

The mean ODD testing scores were 0.79 ± 0.25 for the images in the ODD testing group and 0.10 ± 0.12 in the healthy control group. The mean healthy testing scores were 0.09 ± 0.15 for the images in the ODD testing group and 0.90 ± 0.12 for the healthy control group.

The difference between the mean testing scores for the differentiation of diseased and healthy optic discs was statistically significant ($p < 0.001$) for both FAF and CFP images.

3.3. Repeatability and Precision

The initial computed testing scores and the scores of the repeated testing had a mean coefficient of variation of $0.22 \pm 0.59\%$ (FAF) and $3.73 \pm 5.83\%$ (CFP), respectively, indicating both classifiers had good precision. Between the two tests, the mean difference had absolute values of 0.001 ± 0.005 (FAF) and 0.006 ± 0.07 (CFP).

The Bland–Altman plots indicate high values of repeatability for both classifiers. The results for the classifier using FAF images were even superior to that using CFP images, as seen in Figure 3.

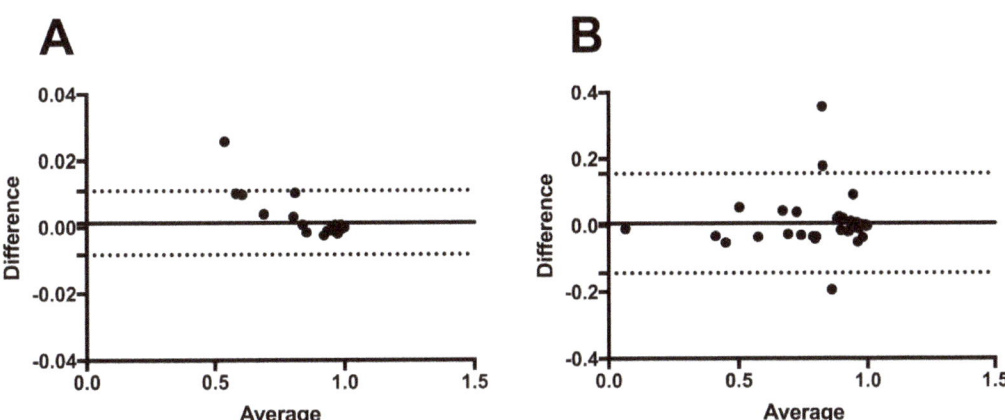

Figure 3. To determine the degree of agreement between the test results from the initial and subsequent deep learning procedures using fundus autofluorescence (**A**) and color fundus photography (**B**), Bland–Altman plots were used. The average difference in ODD score between the two treatments is shown by the solid line. The ranges ([mean of the difference] + 1.96 [standard deviation of the difference]) and ([mean of the difference] − 1.96 [standard deviation of the difference]) are shown by the dashed lines.

4. Discussion

Machine learning (ML) and deep learning (DL) have increased the possibilities for automatic image analysis in ophthalmology. DL has been successfully used for the automatic detection of diseases with high prevalence, such as diabetic retinopathy [18,29], age-related macular degeneration [27,30], and glaucoma [17], using different image modalities. In this context, it seems plausible to extend the use of DL to other, less frequent diseases, like optic disc drusen (ODD). Our results show that DL is a suitable approach to facilitate image analysis in this rare diagnosis.

Many of the DL studies mentioned above achieved a sensitivity and specificity of more than 90%, but in most of them, thousands of images were necessary to train the algorithms [17,18,27]. Despite the small amount of data used due to the low prevalence of ODD, especially when compared to widespread diseases, the classifiers used in this study achieved an accuracy of 100% and 92.5%, respectively. Additionally, this approach has already been successfully applied in pre-published work [27,28,31].

Shah et al. were able to show in a preliminary study that DL can be effectively used with a small amount of data for training to classify normal OCT scans and those from patients with Stargardt's disease at different stages and, therefore, characteristic of the disease [32]. Training and testing data were composed of 749 OCT B-scans of only 93 individuals. Similar to our study, a CNN architecture pre-trained with the ImageNet dataset was used and achieved sensitivity and specificity levels of over 95% [26].

In our study, an even smaller amount of FAF and CFP images was used, achieving similar results with a sensitivity of 100% for both classifiers and a specificity of 100% with fundus autofluorescence and 85% with color fundus imaging.

Different aspects could explain why a similar performance of the algorithm was achieved in this study although an even smaller data set was used.

First, the use of multiple images of a single eye potentially reduced the diversity within the data set of Shah et al. [32]. In our study, only one image of a single eye was used. Second, the use of data from one disease at various stages of Stargardt's disease leads to a limited ability of the classification model to differentiate images with a milder disease phenotype. In contrast, our study only considered images with superficial drusen. This makes it easier for the algorithm to learn specific aspects of this disease subgroup, although its field of application is limited to a smaller patient collective.

In our study, we used FAF and CFP images to analyze ODD because first, superficial ODD visible in FAF have a higher risk of causing a visual field defect compared to buried ODD [11], and second, CFP imaging is a widely used image modality in screening examinations. Thus, the algorithm could be used as s screening tool for visible ODD on color fundus photographs to then initiate further diagnostics, such as performing a visual field examination.

Comparing the results of FAF and CFP image analysis, patterns of ODD seemed to be easier to recognize on FAF images for the algorithm. This can be seen in the relatively flatter training accuracy curve in Figure 2 and is an indicator of a higher learning rate. Additionally, the DCNN is able to distinguish more clearly between healthy subjects and ODD on FAF images. All ODD eyes were correctly identified on FAF images, whereas three CFP images were misdiagnosed as being healthy (Figure 4). This may indicate that FAF is superior to CFP in the identification of superficial optic disc drusen. This seems plausible since visible drusen in FAF are clearly distinguishable by autofluorescence [7].

However, RGB images (CFP) are 3-channel color images, while greyscale images (FAF) have only one channel that represents the intensity of the image. When using InceptionV3, the model would expect an input image with the same number of channels as its pre-trained weights. If a grayscale image is fed as an input, it would have to be first converted to an RGP image by repeating the single channel across the three channels. Thus, it could be expected that the DCNN might perform better when given RGB images as input compared to grayscale images. However, if the FAF images contain sufficient information for the task, they may even outperform RGB images, which is the case in our study [33].

Three CFB images were misdiagnosed by the classifier (Figure 4). Due to the black box formation of DCNN the reasons for misdiagnosis of the images by the classifier can only be suspected. However, one reason for this could be that in these three cases, the drusen are not clearly delineated on fundus photographs despite their visibility in fundus autofluorescence.

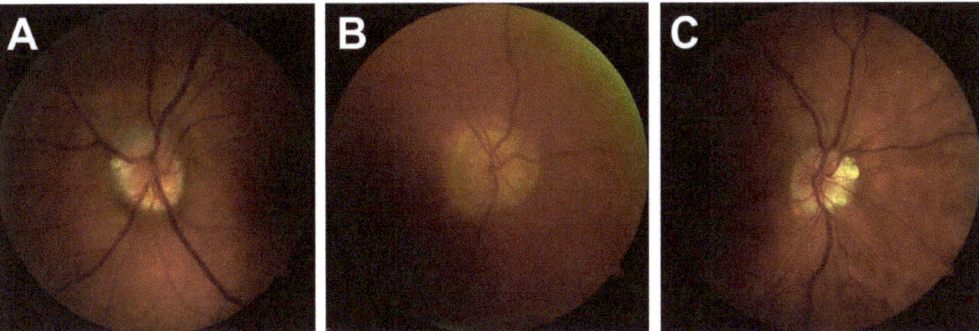

Figure 4. Three ODD images were incorrectly identified as healthy optic discs. This might be due to (**A**) low contrast according to the Juvenile reflexes and mostly buried optic discs drusen, (**B**) low contrast due to low image quality, (**C**) unclear.

Even though the applicability for FAF images was better, the CFP images analysis also showed promising results. Automated analysis of CFP images will probably play an even more important role in everyday clinical routine. In contrast to FAF, CFP imaging is a widespread procedure in screening, even without symptoms, in many in- and outpatient settings. The increasing usefulness of fundus imaging offers a vast amount of data that clinicians must thoroughly assess quickly. Similar to computer-assisted detection systems created to help radiologists interpret medical pictures, DL methods, as applied in this study, could help radiologists with the diagnosis and treatment of optic disc illnesses [14]. This could increase the usefulness of screening examinations in general and help to ensure that the data collected are actually fully evaluated and a true benefit for the patient can be derived.

In a recent study, Milea et al. used a deep learning system to detect papilledema on color fundus photographs using a dataset of 14,341 images. They reached sensitivity levels of 96.4% and specificity of 84.7% [34]. Here, ODD were analyzed as a part of a group of "Disks with Other Abnormalities" and were, therefore, not discussed separately. However, the performance results of the algorithms are comparable [34].

This study was limited by different aspects. First, by training the DCNNs exclusively with visible ODD, the algorithms presented here have questionable relevance to everyday clinical practice. For an ophthalmologist, detecting visible ODD, especially using FAF images, is, in most cases, very simple. Therefore, the high specificity and sensitivity values achieved here are not surprising. In contrast, the detection of buried optic disc drusen and its differentiation from other optic disc pathologies, such as optic disc edema, is both highly clinically significant and challenging. In order to support ophthalmologists in their decision-making based on artificial intelligence in everyday clinical practice, further studies are necessary, including buried optic disc drusen. In this pilot study, however, the primary aim was to detect superficial drusen. The classification of deep ODD and its differentiation from other optic nerve pathologies is planned in a follow-up study.

Second, each of our DL classifiers was trained and tested on FAF and CFP images from a single device type. Therefore, the applicability to FAF and CFP images from other devices is unknown. However, we believe that image data from different devices can be used after prior alignment to uniform recording conditions.

Third, the image data set for this study was small compared to other AI studies in the field of ophthalmology. However, as explained above, this can also be seen as a strength of our approach since it can be difficult and time-consuming to build up large data pools, especially for rare diseases. Therefore, algorithms that make reliable statements based on smaller data sets offer an exciting perspective. Maybe, the results of our testing will even improve with a higher amount of data.

Finally, overfitting is a risk associated with using a small dataset to train a DCNN. This can happen if the model is trained with only a few images or with a large number of training steps. The risk is that the model corresponds too closely to the training data and fails to make reliable predictions on new data. In other words, the model is learning patterns that are unique to the training data but irrelevant to other data. The capacity of the DCNN to detect unseen images decreases with subsequent training steps after an initial improvement. Based on the training and validation accuracy curves, an increasing gap is formed between the training and validation accuracy curves. There were no significant differences in the course of the curves of training and validation accuracy in this study, indicating that neither model is overfitting.

5. Conclusions

In conclusion, we were able to demonstrate that it is possible to use DL classification models to differentiate between normal FAF and CFP images and those from patients with superficial ODD using a transfer-learning-based DL algorithm.

FAF images seem to be superior to CFP images in the diagnostics using our DL approach. However, the analysis of CFP images also showed promising results. Prospective studies will be crucial for clinical translation and will hopefully confirm and improve our results.

We hypothesize that the general principle demonstrated in this study can be applied to other optic disc abnormalities with a lower prevalence.

Author Contributions: Conceptualization, R.D. and M.T.; methodology, R.D. and M.T.; software, M.T.; validation, R.D., J.L.L. and M.T.; formal analysis, R.D., J.L.L., N.E. and M.T.; resources, N.E.; data curation, R.D.; writing—original draft preparation, R.D.; writing—review and editing, J.L.L., N.E. and M.T.; visualization, R.D., J.L.L.; supervision, N.E.; project administration, M.T. All authors have read and agreed to the published version of the manuscript.

Funding: This research received no external funding.

Institutional Review Board Statement: The study was conducted in accordance with the Declaration of Helsinki and adhered to the ethical standards issued by the ethics committee of the Westphalian Wilhelms-University of Münster, Germany. Ethical review and approval was waived for this study due to its retrospective nature and the use of a fully anonymized dataset.

Informed Consent Statement: Patient consent was waived due to the retrospective nature of this study and the use of a fully anonymized dataset.

Data Availability Statement: Not applicable.

Conflicts of Interest: The authors declare no conflict of interest.

References

1. Auw-Haedrich, C.; Staubach, F.; Witschel, H. Optic disk drusen. *Surv. Ophthalmol.* **2002**, *47*, 515–532. [CrossRef] [PubMed]
2. Lorentzen, S.E. Drusen of the optic disk. A clinical and genetic study. *Acta Ophthalmol.* **1996**, *90*, 1–180.
3. Baehring, J.M.; Biestek, J.S. Optic nerve head Drusen mimicking papilledema. *J. Neuro-Oncol.* **2005**, *72*, 47. [CrossRef] [PubMed]
4. Hu, K.; Davis, A.; O'Sullivan, E. Distinguishing optic disc drusen from papilloedema. *BMJ* **2008**, *337*, a2360. [CrossRef]
5. Palmer, E.; Gale, J.; Crowston, J.G.; Wells, A.P. Optic Nerve Head Drusen: An Update. *Neuro-Ophthalmol.* **2018**, *42*, 367–384. [CrossRef]
6. Sim, P.Y.; Soomro, H.; Karampelas, M.; Barampouti, F. Enhanced Depth Imaging Optical Coherence Tomography of Optic Nerve Head Drusen in Children. *J. Neuro-Ophthalmol.* **2020**, *40*, 498–503. [CrossRef]
7. Hamann, S.; Malmqvist, L.; Costello, F. Optic disc drusen: Understanding an old problem from a new perspective. *Acta Ophthalmol.* **2018**, *96*, 673–684. [CrossRef]
8. Savino, P.J.; Glaser, J.S.; Rosenberg, M.A. A Clinical Analysis of Pseudopapilledema: II. Visual Field Defects. *Arch. Ophthalmol.* **1979**, *97*, 71–75. [CrossRef]
9. Mustonen, E. Pseudopapilloedema with and without verified optic disc drusen. A clinical analysis II: Visual fields. *Acta Ophthalmol.* **1983**, *61*, 1057–1066. [CrossRef]
10. Mistlberger, A.; Sitte, S.; Hommer, A.; Emesz, M.; Dengg, S.; Hitzl, W.; Grabner, G. Scanning Laser Polarimetry (SLP) for Optic Nerve Head Drusen. *Int. Ophthalmol.* **2001**, *23*, 233–237. [CrossRef]

11. Malmqvist, L.; Wegener, M.; Sander, B.A.; Hamann, S. Peripapillary Retinal Nerve Fiber Layer Thickness Corresponds to Drusen Location and Extent of Visual Field Defects in Superficial and Buried Optic Disc Drusen. *J. Neuro-Ophthalmol.* **2016**, *36*, 41–45. [CrossRef]
12. LeCun, Y.; Bengio, Y.; Hinton, G. Deep learning. *Nature* **2015**, *521*, 436–444. [CrossRef]
13. Hekler, A.; Utikal, J.S.; Enk, A.H.; Solass, W.; Schmitt, M.; Klode, J.; Schadendorf, D.; Sondermann, W.; Franklin, C.; Bestvater, F.; et al. Deep learning outperformed 11 pathologists in the classification of histopathological melanoma images. *Eur. J. Cancer* **2019**, *118*, 91–96. [CrossRef]
14. McBee, M.P.; Awan, O.A.; Colucci, A.T.; Ghobadi, C.W.; Kadom, N.; Kansagra, A.P.; Tridandapani, S.; Auffermann, W.F. Deep Learning in Radiology. *Acad. Radiol.* **2018**, *25*, 1472–1480. [CrossRef]
15. Wang, S.; Yang, D.M.; Rong, R.; Zhan, X.; Xiao, G. Pathology Image Analysis Using Segmentation Deep Learning Algorithms. *Am. J. Pathol.* **2019**, *189*, 1686–1698. [CrossRef]
16. Ting, D.S.; Peng, L.; Varadarajan, A.V.; Keane, P.A.; Burlina, P.M.; Chiang, M.F.; Schmetterer, L.; Pasquale, L.R.; Bressler, N.M.; Webster, D.R.; et al. Deep learning in ophthalmology: The technical and clinical considerations. *Prog. Retin. Eye Res.* **2019**, *72*, 100759. [CrossRef]
17. Li, F.; Yan, L.; Wang, Y.; Shi, J.; Chen, H.; Zhang, X.; Jiang, M.; Wu, Z.; Zhou, K. Deep learning-based automated detection of glaucomatous optic neuropathy on color fundus photographs. *Graefe's Arch. Clin. Exp. Ophthalmol.* **2020**, *258*, 851–867. [CrossRef]
18. Gulshan, V.; Peng, L.; Coram, M.; Stumpe, M.C.; Wu, D.; Narayanaswamy, A.; Venugopalan, S.; Widner, K.; Madams, T.; Cuadros, J.; et al. Development and Validation of a Deep Learning Algorithm for Detection of Diabetic Retinopathy in Retinal Fundus Photographs. *JAMA* **2016**, *316*, 2402–2410. [CrossRef]
19. Peng, Y.; Dharssi, S.; Chen, Q.; Keenan, T.D.; Agrón, E.; Wong, W.T.; Chew, E.Y.; Lu, Z. DeepSeeNet: A Deep Learning Model for Automated Classification of Patient-based Age-related Macular Degeneration Severity from Color Fundus Photographs. *Ophthalmology* **2018**, *126*, 565–575. [CrossRef]
20. Angermueller, C.; Pärnamaa, T.; Parts, L.; Stegle, O. Deep learning for computational biology. *Mol. Syst. Biol.* **2016**, *12*, 878. [CrossRef]
21. Treder, M.; Eter, N. Deep Learning" und neuronale Netzwerke in der Augenheilkunde. *Ophthalmologe* **2018**, *115*, 714–721. [CrossRef] [PubMed]
22. Szegedy, C.; Vanhoucke, V.; Ioffe, S.; Shlens, J.; Wojna, Z. Rethinking the Inception Architecture for Computer Vision. In Proceedings of the IEEE Conference on Computer Vision and Pattern Recognition (CVPR), Las Vegas, NV, USA, 27–30 June 2016; pp. 2818–2826.
23. Chen, T.; Li, M.; Li, Y.; Lin, M.; Wang, N.; Wang, M.; Xiao, T.; Xu, B.; Zhang, C.; Zhang, Z. TensorFlow: Large-scale machine learning on heterogeneous distributed systems. *arXiv* **2015**, arXiv:1512.01274. Available online: https://static.googleusercontent.com/media/research.google.com/en//pubs/archive/45166.pdf (accessed on 4 June 2017).
24. TensorFlow. 2017. Available online: http://www.tensorflow.org/tutorials/image_recognition (accessed on 26 June 2017).
25. Google Developers. 2017. Available online: https://codelabs.developers.google/.com/codelabs/tensorflow-for-poets/#0 (accessed on 4 July 2017).
26. Deng, J.; Dong, W.; Socher, R.; Li, L.J.; Li, K.; Fei-Fei, L. ImageNet: A large-scale hierarchical image database. In Proceedings of the IEEE Conference on Computer Vision and Pattern Recognition, Miami, FL, USA, 16–20 June 2009; pp. 248–255.
27. Treder, M.; Lauermann, J.L.; Eter, N. Automated detection of exudative age-related macular degeneration in spectral domain optical coherence tomography using deep learning. *Graefe's Arch. Clin. Exp. Ophthalmol.* **2017**, *256*, 259–265. [CrossRef] [PubMed]
28. Treder, M.; Lauermann, J.L.; Eter, N. Deep learning-based detection and classification of geographic atrophy using a deep convolutional neural network classifier. *Graefe's Arch. Clin. Exp. Ophthalmol.* **2018**, *256*, 2053–2060. [CrossRef] [PubMed]
29. Raman, R.; Srinivasan, S.; Virmani, S.; Sivaprasad, S.; Rao, C.; Rajalakshmi, R. Fundus photograph-based deep learning algorithms in detecting diabetic retinopathy. *Eye* **2018**, *33*, 97–109. [CrossRef]
30. Burlina, P.M.; Joshi, N.; Pekala, M.; Pacheco, K.D.; Freund, D.E.; Bressler, N.M. Automated Grading of Age-Related Macular Degeneration From Color Fundus Images Using Deep Convolutional Neural Networks. *JAMA Ophthalmol.* **2017**, *135*, 1170–1176. [CrossRef]
31. Treder, M.; Lauermann, J.L.; Alnawaiseh, M.; Eter, N. Using Deep Learning in Automated Detection of Graft Detachment in Descemet Membrane Endothelial Keratoplasty: A Pilot Study. *Cornea* **2018**, *38*, 157–161. [CrossRef]
32. Shah, M.; Ledo, A.R.; Rittscher, J. Automated classification of normal and Stargardt disease optical coherence tomography images using deep learning. *Acta Ophthalmol.* **2020**, *98*, e715–e721. [CrossRef]
33. Krizhevsky, A.; Sutskever, I.; Hinton, G.E. Imagenet classification with deep convolutional neural networks. *Commun. ACM* **2017**, *60*, 84–90. [CrossRef]
34. Milea, D.; Najjar, R.P.; Jiang, Z.; Ting, D.; Vasseneix, C.; Xu, X.; Fard, M.A.; Fonseca, P.; Vanikieti, K.; Lagrèze, W.A.; et al. Artificial Intelligence to Detect Papilledema from Ocular Fundus Photographs. *N. Engl. J. Med.* **2020**, *382*, 1687–1695. [CrossRef]

Disclaimer/Publisher's Note: The statements, opinions and data contained in all publications are solely those of the individual author(s) and contributor(s) and not of MDPI and/or the editor(s). MDPI and/or the editor(s) disclaim responsibility for any injury to people or property resulting from any ideas, methods, instructions or products referred to in the content.

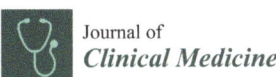

Article

En Face Choroidal Vascularity in Both Eyes of Patients with Unilateral Central Serous Chorioretinopathy

Filippo Tatti [1], Claudio Iovino [1,2], Giuseppe Demarinis [1], Emanuele Siotto Pintor [1], Marco Pellegrini [3], Oliver Beale [4], Kiran Kumar Vupparaboina [4], Mohammed Abdul Rasheed [5], Giuseppe Giannaccare [3,6], Jay Chhablani [4] and Enrico Peiretti [1,*]

1. Eye Clinic, Department of Surgical Sciences, University of Cagliari, 09124 Cagliari, Italy
2. Eye Clinic, Multidisciplinary Department of Medical, Surgical and Dental Sciences, University of Campania Luigi Vanvitelli, 80131 Naples, Italy
3. Ophthalmology Unit, S. Orsola-Malpighi University Hospital, University of Bologna, 40138 Bologna, Italy
4. Department of Ophthalmology, University of Pittsburgh, Pittsburgh, PA 15213, USA
5. School of Optometry and Vision Science, University of Waterloo, Waterloo, ON N2L 3G1, Canada
6. Department of Ophthalmology, University "Magna Graecia", 88100 Catanzaro, Italy
* Correspondence: enripei@hotmail.com

Abstract: The aim of this study was to evaluate the choroidal vascularity analyzing en face optical coherence tomography (OCT) images in patients with unilateral central serous chorioretinopathy (CSC). We retrospectively evaluated 40 eyes of 20 CSC patients and 20 eyes of 10 gender- and age-matched healthy individuals. The sample consisted of: (1) CSC affected eyes; (2) unaffected fellow eyes; (3) healthy eyes. Multiple cross-sectional enhanced depth imaging OCT scans were obtained to create a volume scan. En face scans of the whole choroid were obtained at 5µm intervals and were binarized to calculate the choroidal vascularity index (CVI). The latter, defined as the proportion of the luminal area to the total choroidal area, was calculated at the level of choriocapillaris, superficial, medium and deep layers. No significant differences between choriocapillaris, superficial, medium and deep CVI were found in both eyes of CSC patients, whereas a significant different trend of changes was found in healthy eyes. Nevertheless, the en face CVI shows no difference between affected fellow and healthy eyes. In conclusion, CSC-affected eyes and fellow eyes showed a similar vascular architecture, with no statistical difference between all choroidal layers.

Keywords: central serous chorioretinopathy; pachychoroid; en face optical coherence tomography; choroid; choroidal vascularity index

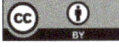

1. Introduction

Central serous chorioretinopathy (CSC) is characterized by localized serous detachment of the neurosensory retina, with or without focal detachments or alterations of the retinal pigment epithelium (RPE) [1,2]. This disorder, mostly seen in young and middle-aged males, typically is self-limited, but it may recur or persist in the chronic form of the disease [1]. Although CSC usually manifests in one eye, it may occur as a bilateral condition. Under this light, in the literature, the incidence of bilateral CSC at the initial visit is reported to be between 5% to 18% [3], whereas a bilateral involvement was found to increase with a longer follow-up [3–6].

The alteration of the choroidal vasculature is a well-known factor in the pathogenesis of CSC [7]. The choroidal involvement was firstly demonstrated by the features on an indocyanine angiography (ICGA), such as hyperpermeable dilated choroidal vessels [8], and this is considered a hallmark of the disease. However, while the ICGA is able to better delineate the choroidal vessels, it does not allow to localize the vascular features in their respective tissue layers [9–11]. Therefore the optical coherence tomography (OCT) development and the introduction of novel imaging techniques, such as enhanced-depth imaging (EDI) and swept source (SS), have facilitated the detailed and depth-resolved evaluation of the choroidal morphology in CSC patients [12–14].

Additionally, a choroidal vasculature evaluation in CSC patients was obtained using the choroidal vascularity index (CVI), a new parameter defined as the ratio between the luminal choroidal area (LCA) and the total choroidal area (TCA) on OCT B-scans [15–18]. In a recent study, this parameter allowed to show an increased vascular component compared with the stromal component in eyes affected by CSC. Indeed, an increased choroidal vascularity index was demonstrated in affected eyes compared with fellow ones. However, fellow eyes also showed a higher CVI in comparison with age-matched healthy subjects. As previously reported, the CVI could then be a useful index for early diagnosis of CSC and the assessment of the treatment response after photodynamic therapy [16,17].

Nevertheless, the CVI measured on the foveal cross-sectional B-scan cannot reveal the overall picture of the choroidal status [19–21]. For this reason, the CVI has been recently measured also on en face OCT scans to obtain a more real representation of the choroidal vasculature in healthy or affected eyes [22,23]. The en face CVI evaluation at various levels of the choroid showed a similar trend of changes in acute and chronic CSC patients [23].

The aim of the present study was to evaluate the CVI changes in both eyes of patients with unilateral CSC by analyzing en face OCT images generated through volumetric maps.

2. Materials and Methods

A consecutive series of 20 patients with diagnoses of unilateral CSC were evaluated in this retrospective study. All subjects were attended to at the Retina Center of the Eye Clinic, University of Cagliari. The study adhered to the tenets of the Declaration of Helsinki and the protocol used was approved by the local Institutional Review Board (NP/2022/3119). A complete ophthalmic examination was performed for each patient, including Snellen best-corrected visual acuity (BCVA), fundus autofluorescence, fluorescein angiography (FA) and ICGA (Heidelberg Spectralis, Heidelberg Engineering), intraocular pressure (IOP) measurement, anterior segment and fundus examination. Unilateral CSC was defined as a prior or active unilateral manifestation of CSC. Thus, patients evidencing any presence or evidence of previous subretinal fluid in the fellow eyes were excluded from the study. The exclusion criteria were also refractive error >±3, macular pathologies other than CSC, as well as the presence of MNV and any ocular surgery. Patients with a history of any treatment in the previous 3 months and of any previous treatment that could affect CVI were also excluded [24,25]. A history of any previous medications that could cause subretinal fluid was also recorded. The patient group was compared with a gender- and age-matched control group (20 eyes of 10 healthy individuals).

2.1. Spectral-Domain Optical Coherence Tomography Analysis

For each eye, a posterior pole volumetric scan containing multiple high density cross-sectional scans (49B, 30 × 20°) was obtained using the spectral-domain (SD) OCT with EDI mode. The scans were obtained for each patient in the afternoon at the set time frame 2–4 pm. These data were exported from the Heidelberg device as images with a 1:1 pixel ratio.

Central macular thickness (CMT) was defined as the average thickness of a 1 mm diameter circle centered on the foveal center, measuring from the internal limiting membrane and the RPE. Subfoveal choroidal thickness (CT) was obtained by measuring the distance between RPE–Bruch's membrane complex and the choroidoscleral interface.

2.2. Choroidal En Face OCT Extraction

The algorithm involved in obtaining the en face CVI measurement included the choroidal en face OCT extraction and the binarization of the en face OCT scans, following an already tested procedure [22].

The choroid was firstly segmented from the OCT volume. In particular, each B-scan of the volume scan was analyzed to segment choroid on a previously validated algorithm where the RPE–Bruch's membrane complex and the CSI were identified using structural similarity (SSIM), Hessian analysis and tensor voting [26]. Segmented choroidal sections were subsequently stacked to obtain the choroid volume, and multiple 5 micron spacing en face sections were generated for the CVI analysis.

2.3. En Face CVI estimation

Adaptive histogram equalization was employed (using a built in MATLAB v2018b function) in order to increase the contrast between choroidal vessel lumen and the stroma. Blood vessels were then separated using the block-based particle swarm optimization (PSO) thresholding [22,27]. The binarized images were reviewed by two independent observers blinded to each other to assess whether the images were correctly converted by comparing with the original en face OCT images. This process was performed twice for each image by each observer.

CVI was calculated for every en face image separated by 5 µm within the choroid volume. The layer of small choroidal vessels, including choriocapillaris, was defined as a dense network of small vessels just 10 µm beneath Bruch's membrane.

The points of measurements were manually identified in each eye, focusing on major anatomical locations (i.e., Bruch's membrane, choriocapillaris and choroidoscleral interface) and at various depths from RPE–Bruch's membrane complex. The maximum choroidal thickness across the volume cube was divided by three (superficial or inner layer, medium and deep or outer layer) for both eyes. Hence, the mean CVI was calculated for the choriocapillaris, the inner/superficial third, the middle/medium third and the outer/deep third of the choroidal thickness. (Figures 1 and 2).

2.4. Statistical Analysis

The statistical analysis was conducted with R (version 4.0.0) and RStudio (version 1.2.5042) software. The Kolmogorov–Smirnov test was used to evaluate the normal distribution for each variable. The CVI was compared between CSC eyes and fellow eyes by using paired samples t-test or Wilcoxon test. A repeated measures ANOVA or Friedman test was used to compare the choroidal vascularity of choriocapillaris, superficial, medium and deep third of the choroid. A p value < 0.05 was considered statistically significant.

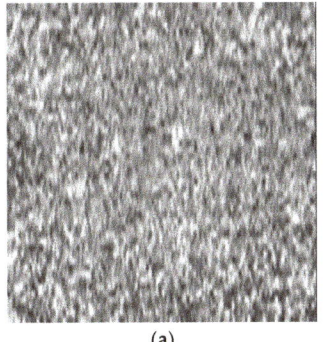
(a)

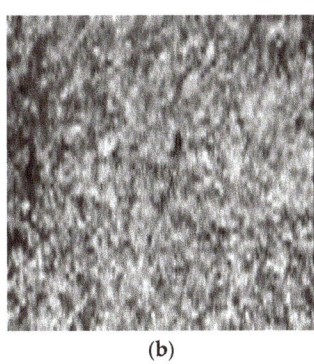
(b)

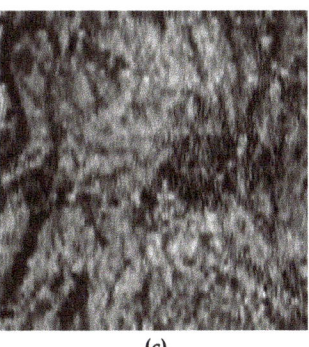
(c)

Figure 1. *Cont.*

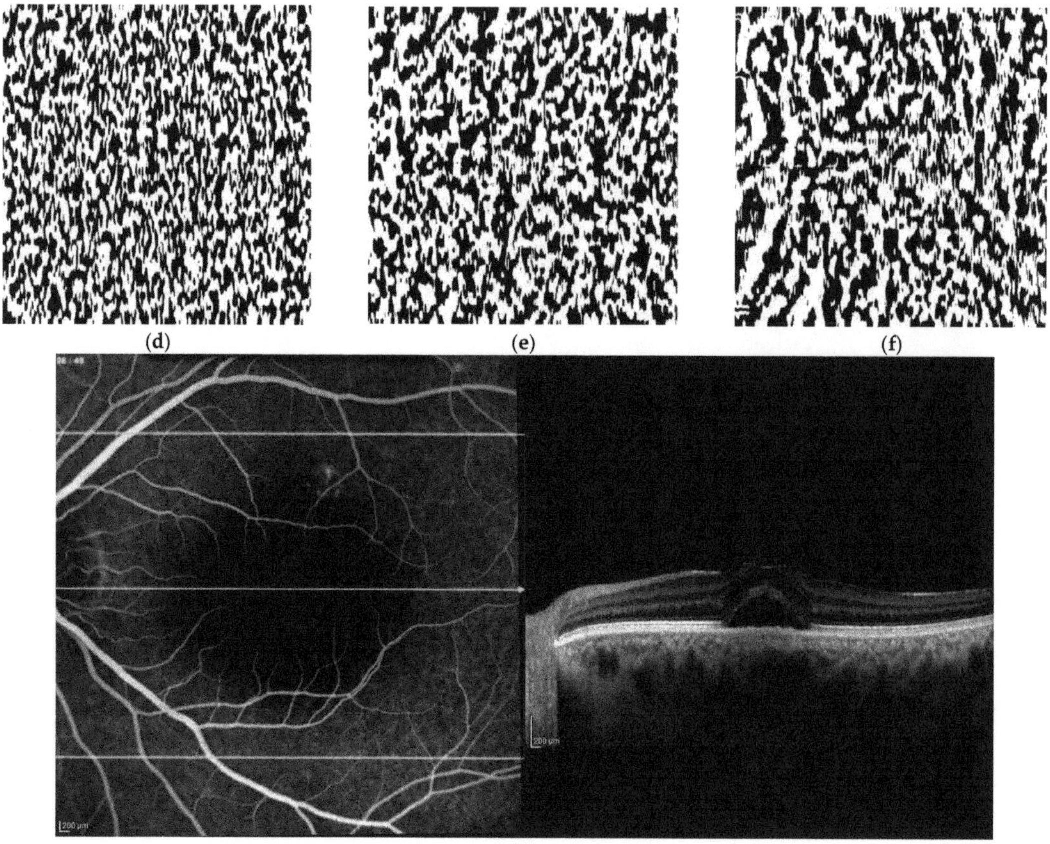

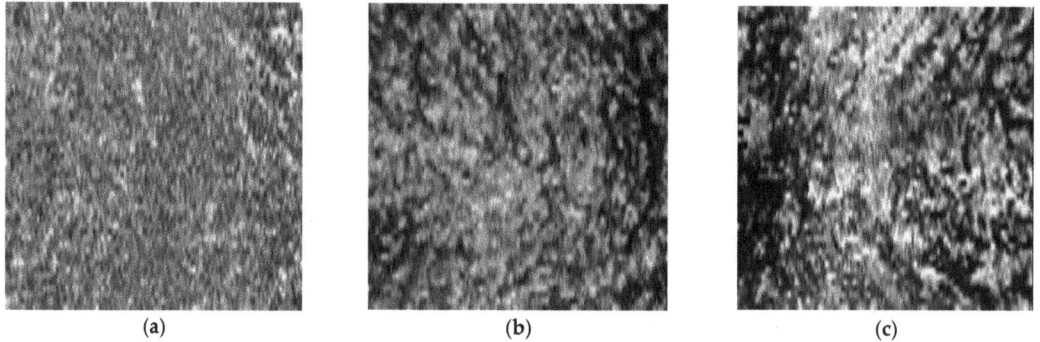

Figure 1. Original en face optical coherence tomography (OCT) scans and the software-processed images of an affected eye of a patient with central serous chorioretinopathy. Original en face OCT scan images of the superficial (**a**), medium (**b**) and deep (**c**) choroidal layer; binarized images of the superficial (**d**), medium (**e**) and deep (**f**) choroidal layer; OCT B-scan across the foveal center (**g**).

Figure 2. *Cont.*

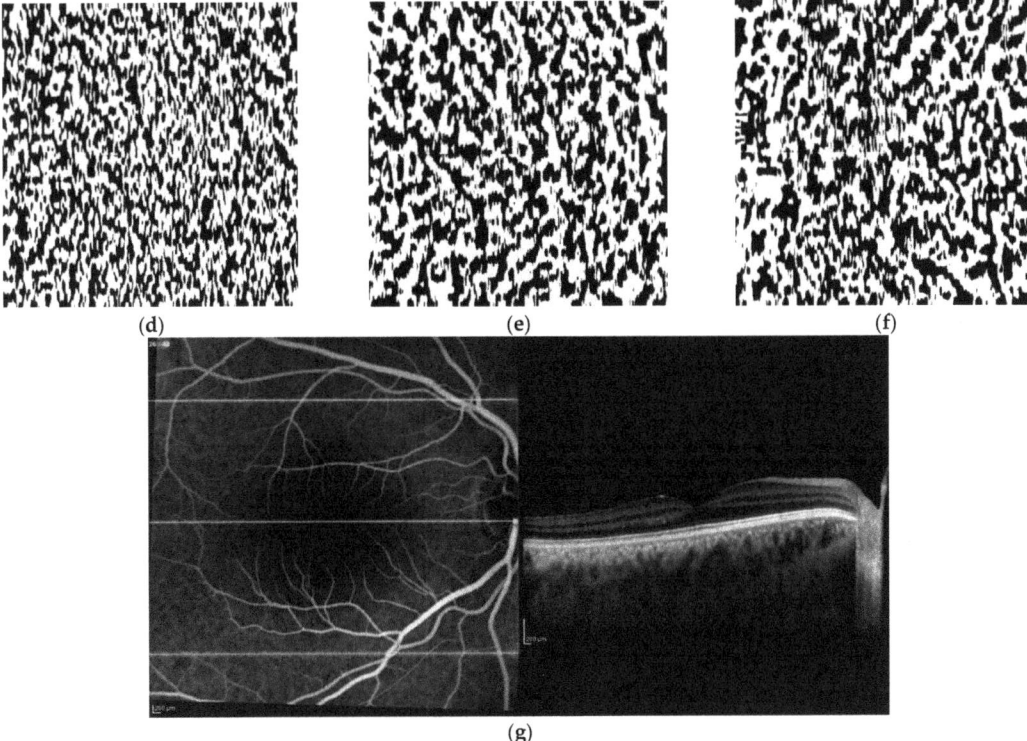

Figure 2. Original en face optical coherence tomography (OCT) scans and the software-processed images of the fellow eye of the same patient of Figure 1. Original en face OCT scan images of the superficial (**a**), medium (**b**) and deep (**c**) choroidal layer; binarized images of the superficial (**d**), medium (**e**) and deep (**f**) choroidal layer; OCT B-scan across the foveal center (**g**).

3. Results

A total of 20 patients (16 males and 4 females) were included. The average age was 50.7 ± 9.96 years. The average BCVA was 0.28 ± 0.35 logMAR for CSC eyes and 0.03 ± 0.09 logMAR for fellow eyes. Previous treatments included only nonsteroidal anti-inflammatory drugs (10 patients). The average time between the diagnosis and the evaluation was 2.42 ± 2.47 years.

The gender- and age-matched control group included 20 eyes of 10 individuals (eight males and two females) with a mean age of 48.8 ± 3.5 years. The demographic data showed no statistical difference with the study group (all $p > 0.05$).

The choroidal parameters in CSC, fellow and healthy eyes are reported in Table 1.

The subfoveal CT was significantly higher in eyes with CSC compared with fellow eyes (489.8 ± 13.4 vs. 433.7 ± 12.2; $p = 0.047$). The first third segment thickness resulted on average 163.3 ± 44.8 μm and 144.6 ± 41.6 μm for affected eyes and fellow eyes, respectively. Consecutively, these values represented the average thicknesses of the choroidal segments. For the average en face CVI, no significant difference between the CSC and fellow eyes was observed ($p = 0.681$). Similarly, no significant differences in the choriocapillaris, superficial, medium and deep CVI were found (respectively, $p = 0.940$, $p = 0.685$ and $p = 0.411$; $p = 0.627$) (Table 1).

Table 1. Choroidal parameters in eyes with CSC, fellow and healthy eyes.

Parameter (Mean ± SD)	CSC Eyes (20)	Fellow Eyes (20)	CSC vs. Fellow Eyes (p)	Healthy Eyes (20)	CSC vs. Healthy Eyes (p)	Fellow vs. Healthy Eyes (p)
Subfoveal CT (μm)	489.8 ± 13.4	433.7 ± 12.2	0.047	334 ± 58.2	<0.01	<0.01
Whole CVI	0.494 ± 0.045	0.484 ± 0.044	0.681	0.488 ± 0.002	0.372	0.955
Choriocapillaris CVI	0.491 ± 0,082	0.497 ± 0.060	0.940	0.469 ± 0.004	0.704	0.900
Superficial layer CVI	0.497 ± 0.020	0.500 ± 0.024	0.685	0.506 ± 0,001	0.690	0.273
Medium layer CVI	0.498 ± 0.027	0.490 ± 0.021	0.411	0.492 ± 0.004	0.088	0.370
Deep layer CVI	0.487 ± 0.107	0.463 ± 0.103	0.627	0.506 ± 0.010	0.448	0.081
Choroidal layer comparison (p)	0.73	0.16		<0.01		

CSC—central serous chorioretinopathy; CT—choroidal thickness; CVI—choroidal vascularity index.

There was a significant difference in subfoveal CT between healthy eyes and both eyes of CSC patients. However, with regard to the CVI layers' comparison, no difference was shown in the layer comparison between healthy and CSC or fellow eyes.

Although a different trend of changes between CSC eyes and fellow eyes, choriocapillaris, superficial, medium and deep CVI did not significantly differ for both ($p = 0.73$; $p = 0.16$). On the contrary, healthy eyes showed a significant difference of CVI among the various choroidal layers ($p < 0.01$).

4. Discussion

We studied the CVI changes across the entire depth of the choroid in both eyes of patients affected by unilateral CSC. In the CSC eyes, the CVI increased as the distance from RPE increased to reach a peak (0.500) in the medium depth of choroid and then reduced towards the CSI (0.495). On the contrary, the mean CVI of fellow eyes tended to reduce from RPE to the CSI (0.501; 0.493; 0.467). The control group showed a different trend, with the lowest average vascular density in the medium layer (0.506; 0.492; 0.506).

Previous studies analyzed the CVI changes in healthy eyes, showing the highest average vascular density in the outer level or Haller's layer [19–22]. Sohrab et al. analyzed only three choroidal sections of en face scans and calculated the vessel density on the basis of a preselected threshold of red, green and blue (RGB) intensity. The authors showed a different average vascular density in choriocapillaris (76.5%), Sattler's layer (83.6%) and Haller's layer (87.2%) [19].

In another study with a cohort of 30 healthy eyes, the CVI values were 53.16%, 51.38% and 55.69%, respectively, at the level of choriocapillaris, medium choroidal vessel and large choroidal vessel layers [22].

The en face CVI of patients affected by acute or chronic CSC was noted to increase as the distance from Bruch's membrane increased. Patients with acute CSC had the point of maximum vascularity (48.35% ± 2.06%) at 75% depth of CT, while those with chronic CSC reached the peak vascularity level at 50% of the choroidal depth, with a CVI of 48.70% ± 1.32% [23].

In our cohort, the variation in CVI between choriocapillaris, superficial, medium and deep level of the choroid were not significant for both eyes. These results are in contrast to those previously reported [23]; a possible reason is the different choroidal segmentation method applied. Indeed, Wong et al. compared choriocapillaris and various choroidal depths of CVI (25%, 33%, 50%, and 75%). Moreover, we have observed no significant difference between the whole and various CVI layers of CSC and fellow eyes, which suggests a similar vascular architecture in both affected and fellow eyes. This could support the theory of a bilateral involvement of CSC, previously revealed by many studies [3–6,8,28–31] and found to increase with a longer follow-up [3–6].

Another aspect to consider is that CSC, as a pachychoroid condition [32], is characterized by an increase in the size of Haller's vessels, which may compress the inner layers and determine a similar vascularity throughout the CT [32,33]. In fact, in severe cases the choriocapillaris and intermediate caliber vessels could be so attenuated that the Haller's layer would occupy a significant proportion of CT [32].

Choroidal thickness analysis suggests that choroidal thickness in eyes with CSC is larger than that in age-matched control eyes and fellow eyes [30,31,34,35]. Considering the multiple factors that could influence the choroidal thickness (age, axial length, refractive error, blood pressure, time of the day), there is no definitive threshold for defining an eye as having pachychoroid [32]. Nevertheless, according to a previous study that considered 395 μm as a sensitive value to diagnose the "pachychoroid" disease, subfoveal CTs of affected and fellow eyes were increased [36].

Interestingly, our study shows how the choroid plays an important role in the pathogenesis of CSC but that it is not the only player. In fact, other than the similar vasculature and the pathological choroidal thickness, there were no signs of CSC in the fellow eye group. In this respect, it is recognized that other factors, such as the RPE, could play defensive roles against high choroidal hydrostatic pressure [37].

The strength of our study is that we provided a measure in vivo of the vascularity across the depth of the choroid, showing some similarities and differences between study eyes and fellow eyes of patients affected by CSC. The study had several weaknesses. First, was the small sample size; indeed, the strict criteria for unilaterality of the disease led to the exclusion of many cases. Considering this limitation, the research should be considered as just a preliminary study that could not provide any definite conclusion. Second, the single time measuring of CVI does not take account of the choroidal variations based on blood pressure and time of day [15]. Lastly, two further limitations arise from the arbitrary cut-offs in identifying the choriocapillaris and the manual identification of the other points of measurement.

5. Conclusions

In this preliminary study, the en face CVI of both eyes of patients affected by CSC showed no difference between affected and fellow eyes. The trend of changes in CVI for CSC and fellow eyes showed no statistical difference in the choroidal layer comparison. On the contrary, healthy eyes showed a significant difference in CVI across the depth of the choroid.

Author Contributions: Conceptualization, C.I., J.C. and E.P.; data curation, O.B., K.K.V. and M.A.R.; formal analysis, M.P. and F.T.; investigation, F.T., G.D., E.S.P., O.B., K.K.V. and M.A.R.; methodology, F.T., C.I. and J.C.; writing—original draft, F.T. and E.P.; writing—review and editing, C.I., G.G., J.C. and E.P. All authors have read and agreed to the published version of the manuscript.

Funding: This research received no external funding.

Institutional Review Board Statement: The study was conducted in accordance with the Declaration of Helsinki, and approved by the Institutional Review Board (or Ethics Committee) of Comitato Etico Indipendente—Azienda Ospedaliero Universitaria di Cagliari (NP/2022/3119).

Informed Consent Statement: Informed consent was obtained from all subjects involved in the study. Written informed consent has been obtained from the patients to publish this paper.

Data Availability Statement: Not applicable.

Conflicts of Interest: The authors declare no conflict of interest.

References

1. Spaide, R.F.; Campeas, L.; Haas, A.; Yannuzzi, L.A.; Fisher, Y.L.; Guyer, D.R.; Slakter, J.S.; Sorenson, J.A.; Orlock, D.A. Central serous chorioretinopathy in younger and older adults. *Ophthalmology* **1996**, *103*, 2070–2080. [CrossRef] [PubMed]
2. Iovino, C.; Chhablani, J.; Parameswarappa, D.C.; Pellegrini, M.; Giannaccare, G.; Peiretti, E. Retinal pigment epithelium apertures as a late complication of longstanding serous pigment epithelium detachments in chronic central serous chorioretinopathy. *Eye* **2019**, *33*, 1871–1876. [CrossRef]

3. Yannuzzi, L.A.; Schatz, H.; Gitter, K.A. Central Serous Chorioretinopathy. In *The Macula: A Comprehensive Text and Atlas*; Williams & Wilkins: Philadelphiam, PA, USA, 1979.
4. Gilbert, C.M.; Owens, S.L.; Smith, P.D.; Fine, S.L. Long-term follow-up of central serous chorioretinopathy. *Br. J. Ophthalmol.* **1984**, *68*, 815–820. [CrossRef] [PubMed]
5. Castro-Correia, J.; Coutinho, M.F.; Rosas, V.; Maia, J. Long-term follow-up of central serous retinopathy in 150 patients. *Doc. Ophthalmol.* **1992**, *81*, 379–386. [CrossRef] [PubMed]
6. Yap, E.Y.; Robertson, D.M. The long-term outcome of central serous chorioretinopathy. *Arch. Ophthalmol.* **1996**, *114*, 689–692. [CrossRef]
7. Mrejen, S.; Spaide, R.F. Optical coherence tomography: Imaging of the choroid and beyond. *Surv. Ophthalmol.* **2013**, *58*, 387–429. [CrossRef]
8. Spaide, R.F.; Hall, L.; Haas, A.; Campeas, L.; Yannuzzi, L.A.; Fisher, Y.L.; Guyer, D.R.; Slakter, J.S.; Sorenson, J.A.; Orlock, D.A. Indocyanine green videoangiography of older patients with central serous chorioretinopathy. *Retina* **1996**, *16*, 203–213. [CrossRef]
9. Yannuzzi, L.A.; Slakter, J.S.; Sorenson, J.A.; Guyer, D.R.; Orlock, D.A. Digital indocyanine green videoangiography and choroidal neovascularization. *Retina* **2012**, *32*, 191. [CrossRef]
10. Klufas, M.A.; Yannuzzi, N.A.; Pang, C.E.; Srinivas, S.; Sadda, S.R.; Freund, K.B.; Kiss, S. Feasibility and clinical utility of ultra-widefield indocyanine green angiography. *Retina* **2015**, *35*, 508–520. [CrossRef]
11. Peiretti, E.; Iovino, C. Chapter 9—Indocyanine Green Angiography. In *Central Serous Chorioretinopathy*; Chhablani, J., Ed.; Academic Press: Cambridge, MA, USA, 2019; pp. 97–113. ISBN 978-0-12-816800-4.
12. Imamura, Y.; Fujiwara, T.; Margolis, R.; Spaide, R.F. Enhanced depth imaging optical coherence tomography of the choroid in central serous chorioretinopathy. *Retina* **2009**, *29*, 1469–1473. [CrossRef]
13. Hamzah, F.; Shinojima, A.; Mori, R.; Yuzawa, M. Choroidal thickness measurement by enhanced depth imaging and swept-source optical coherence tomography in central serous chorioretinopathy. *BMC Ophthalmol.* **2014**, *14*, 145. [CrossRef] [PubMed]
14. Razavi, S.; Souied, E.H.; Cavallero, E.; Weber, M.; Querques, G. Assessment of choroidal topographic changes by swept source optical coherence tomography after photodynamic therapy for central serous chorioretinopathy. *Am. J. Ophthalmol.* **2014**, *157*, 852–860. [CrossRef] [PubMed]
15. Iovino, C.; Pellegrini, M.; Bernabei, F.; Borrelli, E.; Sacconi, R.; Govetto, A.; Vagge, A.; Di Zazzo, A.; Forlini, M.; Finocchio, L.; et al. Choroidal Vascularity Index: An In-Depth Analysis of This Novel Optical Coherence Tomography Parameter. *J. Clin. Med.* **2020**, *9*, 595. [CrossRef] [PubMed]
16. Agrawal, R.; Chhablani, J.; Tan, K.-A.; Shah, S.; Sarvaiya, C.; Banker, A. Choroidal vascularity index in central serous chorioretinopathy. *Retina* **2016**, *36*, 1646–1651. [CrossRef] [PubMed]
17. Iovino, C.; Au, A.; Chhablani, J.; Parameswarappa, D.C.; Rasheed, M.A.; Cennamo, G.; Cennamo, G.; Montorio, D.; Ho, A.C.; Xu, D.; et al. Choroidal Anatomic Alterations After Photodynamic Therapy for Chronic Central Serous Chorioretinopathy: A Multicenter Study. *Am. J. Ophthalmol.* **2020**, *217*, 104–113. [CrossRef]
18. Iovino, C.; Chhablani, J.; Rasheed, M.A.; Tatti, F.; Bernabei, F.; Pellegrini, M.; Giannaccare, G.; Peiretti, E. Effects of different mydriatics on the choroidal vascularity in healthy subjects. *Eye* **2021**, *35*, 913–918. [CrossRef]
19. Sohrab, M.; Wu, K.; Fawzi, A.A. A pilot study of morphometric analysis of choroidal vasculature in vivo, using en face optical coherence tomography. *PLoS ONE* **2012**, *7*, e48631. [CrossRef]
20. Flores-Moreno, I.; Arias-Barquet, L.; Rubio-Caso, M.J.; Ruiz-Moreno, J.M.; Duker, J.S.; Caminal, J.M. En face swept-source optical coherence tomography in neovascular age-related macular degeneration. *Br. J. Ophthalmol.* **2015**, *99*, 1260–1267. [CrossRef]
21. Pilotto, E.; Guidolin, F.; Convento, E.; Antonini, R.; Stefanon, F.G.; Parrozzani, R.; Midena, E. En Face Optical Coherence Tomography to Detect and Measure Geographic Atrophy. *Investig. Ophthalmol. Vis. Sci.* **2015**, *56*, 8120–8124. [CrossRef]
22. Singh, S.R.; Rasheed, M.A.; Parveen, N.; Goud, A.; Ankireddy, S.; Sahoo, N.K.; Vupparaboina, K.K.; Jana, S.; Chhablani, J. En-face choroidal vascularity map of the macula in healthy eyes. *Eur. J. Ophthalmol.* **2021**, *31*, 218–225. [CrossRef]
23. Wong, R.L.-M.; Singh, S.R.; Rasheed, M.A.; Goud, A.; Chhablani, G.; Samantaray, S.; AnkiReddy, S.; Vupparaboina, K.K.; Chhablani, J. En-face choroidal vascularity in central serous chorioretinopathy. *Eur. J. Ophthalmol.* **2020**, *31*, 536–542. [CrossRef] [PubMed]
24. Toto, L.; Ruggeri, M.L.; Evangelista, F.; Viggiano, P.; D'Aloisio, R.; De Nicola, C.; Falconio, G.; Di Nicola, M.; Porreca, A.; Mastropasqua, R. Choroidal modifications assessed by means of choroidal vascularity index after oral eplerenone treatment in chronic central serous chorioretinopathy. *Eye* **2022**. [CrossRef] [PubMed]
25. Park, W.; Kim, M.; Kim, R.Y.; Park, Y.-H. Comparing effects of photodynamic therapy in central serous chorioretinopathy: Full-dose versus half-dose versus half-dose-half-fluence. *Graefe's Arch. Clin. Exp. Ophthalmol. = Albr. Von Graefes Arch. Fur Klin. Exp. Ophthalmol.* **2019**, *257*, 2155–2161. [CrossRef] [PubMed]
26. Vupparaboina, K.K.; Nizampatnam, S.; Chhablani, J.; Richhariya, A.; Jana, S. Automated estimation of choroidal thickness distribution and volume based on OCT images of posterior visual section. *Comput. Med. Imaging Graph. Off. J. Comput. Med. Imaging Soc.* **2015**, *46 Pt 3*, 315–327. [CrossRef]
27. Lahmiri, S.; Boukadoum, M. An Evaluation of Particle Swarm Optimization Techniques in Segmentation of Biomedical Images. In Proceedings of the Companion Publication of the 2014 Annual Conference on Genetic and Evolutionary Computation; Association for Computing Machinery: New York, NY, USA, 2014; pp. 1313–1320.

28. Kim, Y.T.; Kang, S.W.; Bai, K.H. Choroidal thickness in both eyes of patients with unilaterally active central serous chorioretinopathy. *Eye* **2011**, *25*, 1635–1640. [CrossRef] [PubMed]
29. Klein, M.L.; Van Buskirk, E.M.; Friedman, E.; Gragoudas, E.; Chandra, S. Experience with nontreatment of central serous choroidopathy. *Arch. Ophthalmol.* **1974**, *91*, 247–250. [CrossRef]
30. Goktas, A. Correlation of subretinal fluid volume with choroidal thickness and macular volume in acute central serous chorioretinopathy. *Eye* **2014**, *28*, 1431–1436. [CrossRef]
31. Maruko, I.; Iida, T.; Sugano, Y.; Ojima, A.; Sekiryu, T. Subfoveal choroidal thickness in fellow eyes of patients with central serous chorioretinopathy. *Retina* **2011**, *31*, 1603–1608. [CrossRef]
32. Cheung, C.M.G.; Lee, W.K.; Koizumi, H.; Dansingani, K.; Lai, T.Y.Y.; Freund, K.B. Pachychoroid disease. *Eye* **2019**, *33*, 14–33. [CrossRef]
33. Balaratnasingam, C.; Lee, W.-K.; Koizumi, H.; Dansingani, K.; Inoue, M.; Freund, K.B. Polypoidal Choroidal Vasculopathy: A Distinct Disease or Manifestation of Many? *Retina* **2016**, *36*, 1–8. [CrossRef]
34. Oh, J.-H.; Oh, J.; Togloom, A.; Kim, S.-W.; Huh, K. Biometric characteristics of eyes with central serous chorioretinopathy. *Investig. Ophthalmol. Vis. Sci.* **2014**, *55*, 1502–1508. [CrossRef] [PubMed]
35. Yang, L.; Jonas, J.B.; Wei, W. Choroidal vessel diameter in central serous chorioretinopathy. *Acta Ophthalmol.* **2013**, *91*, e358–e362. [CrossRef] [PubMed]
36. Lehmann, M.; Bousquet, E.; Beydoun, T.; Behar-Cohen, F. Pachychoroid: An inherited condition? *Retina* **2015**, *35*, 10–16. [CrossRef] [PubMed]
37. Kaye, R.; Chandra, S.; Sheth, J.; Boon, C.J.F.; Sivaprasad, S.; Lotery, A. Central serous chorioretinopathy: An update on risk factors, pathophysiology and imaging modalities. *Prog. Retin. Eye Res.* **2020**, *79*, 100865. [CrossRef] [PubMed]

Disclaimer/Publisher's Note: The statements, opinions and data contained in all publications are solely those of the individual author(s) and contributor(s) and not of MDPI and/or the editor(s). MDPI and/or the editor(s) disclaim responsibility for any injury to people or property resulting from any ideas, methods, instructions or products referred to in the content.

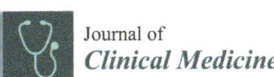

Article

How Could Medical and Surgical Treatment Affect the Quality of Life in Glaucoma Patients? A Cross-Sectional Study

Marco Rocco Pastore [1], Serena Milan [1,*], Rossella Agolini [1], Leonardo Egidi [2], Tiziano Agostini [3], Lorenzo Belfanti [1], Gabriella Cirigliano [1] and Daniele Tognetto [1]

[1] Eye Clinic, Department of Medicine, Surgery and Health Sciences, University of Trieste, 34129 Trieste, Italy
[2] Department of Economics, Business, Mathematics and Statistics, University of Trieste, 34100 Trieste, Italy
[3] Department of Life Sciences, University of Trieste, 34100 Trieste, Italy
* Correspondence: serena.milan2@gmail.com; Tel.: +39-040-399-2243

Abstract: Background: To evaluate and compare the visual function and the quality of life (QoL) in glaucomatous patients treated with topical medical therapy (TMT) alone, canaloplasty (CP), or trabeculectomy (TB). Methods: A total of 291 eyes of 167 patients with primary open-angle glaucoma or secondary pseudoexfoliative glaucoma in TMT or surgically treated with CP or TB were included. Eligibility criteria for surgical patients included not needing TMT after surgery. Each patient underwent a visual field assessment and peripapillary retinal nerve fiber layer (pRNFL) optical coherence tomography and filled out the Glaucoma Symptoms Scale (GSS) questionnaire and the 25-Item National Eye Institute Visual Functioning Questionnaire (25-NEI-VFQ). Comparison between the QoL level of the three groups and its correlation with optic nerve's anatomical and functional status was the primary outcome. Results: CP patients reported the best general vision ($p = 0.01$), a lower incidence of eye burning ($p = 0.03$), and the lowest annoyance level of non-visual symptoms ($p = 0.006$). QoL positively correlated with pRNFL thickness, whereas no correlation was found with visual field damage. Conclusion: CP provides a better QoL when compared both to TB and TMT, regardless of glaucoma stage. pRNFL seems to provide additional information for predicting change in QoL.

Keywords: quality of life; canaloplasty; trabeculectomy; medical therapy

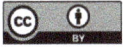

1. Introduction

Glaucoma is a neurodegenerative disease that causes a reduction of chromatic and contrast sensitivity, early alteration of light adaption, and the progressive development of characteristic visual field defects and optic disc damage [1–4]. This condition can lead to difficulties in performing daily activities such as reading, walking, or driving, limiting patients' independence [5,6]. Moreover, the psychological impact can be fairly relevant: the loss of autonomy, together with the fear of going blind, may lead to depression, anxiety, and loneliness [7–9].

The main goal of glaucoma management is to preserve visual function (VF) and quality of life (QoL) [10]. QoL in glaucoma is assuming a leading role in healthcare, representing a significant index of glaucoma impact on patients and of health interventions' effectiveness.

Glaucoma therapeutic options include medical and surgical treatment. Topical medical therapy (TMT) is generally the first approach in reducing intraocular pressure (IOP). However, it can lead to annoying local side effects such as irritation, burning, foreign body sensation, fatigue, blurred vision, dryness, photophobia, dry eye syndrome, allergies, and blepharitis [5,11]. Patients may also have difficulty applying eye drops and following complex treatment regimens. These issues can undermine patients' satisfaction and their compliance with therapy [12,13]. Surgical therapy can reduce the incidence of these side effects; nevertheless, it is associated with specific unpleasant complications. Trabeculectomy

(TB) represents the gold standard in glaucoma surgery, being the most effective surgical procedure for reducing IOP [13]. However, since it implies the creation of a communication between the anterior chamber and the subconjunctival space, it is burdened by numerous intraoperative and postoperative problems such as hypotony, bleb leakage, cataract development, choroidal hemorrhage, and infections [14–16]. Canaloplasty (CP) is a minimally invasive procedure requiring visco-dilatation of the Schlemm's canal and the placement of an intracanalicular tension suture [17]. It has several advantages compared with TB, such as the absence of the filtering bleb and its complications, easier postoperative management, and faster recovery; however, a lower efficacy in reducing IOP was reported [15].

This study aimed to evaluate and compare the VF and the QoL in glaucoma patients treated with TMT, CP, and TB and to correlate it with anatomical and functional optic nerve alterations.

2. Materials and Methods

A cross-sectional study was conducted at the University Eye Clinic of Trieste between October and December 2020. The study protocol adhered to the tenets of the Declaration of Helsinki and was approved by the Institutional Review Board. The nature and the purpose of the investigation were fully explained, and informed consent was obtained from all participants.

Consecutive patients with a diagnosis of primary open angle glaucoma (POAG) or secondary pseudoexfoliative glaucoma (PEXG) in TMT or surgically treated with TB or CP by a single surgeon (DT) between January 2017 and July 2019 were included in the study. Patients were approached by the glaucoma specialist during regular clinic visits and screened for participation in this study. Glaucoma was diagnosed based on the presence of typical glaucomatous optic nerve head damage with focal or generalized neuroretinal rim thinning or cup/disc ratio asymmetry > 2 (in the absence of other neurodegenerative conditions) and associated with repeated corresponding glaucomatous visual field defects. Other eligibility criteria included age ranging between 55 and 80 years, previous cataract surgery, and for surgical patients to have at least 18 months (range, 19–35 months) of postoperative follow-up and no need for TMT after surgery.

Exclusion criteria were previous failed glaucoma surgery (cannulation failure during CP, secondary glaucoma surgery, or IOP > 18 mmHg [18] without topical glaucoma medication), previous eye intervention other than cataract surgery, and the presence of psycho-physical conditions interfering with the comprehension and the compilation of the questionnaires.

Enrolled patients underwent a complete ophthalmic examination and visual field assessment (standard automated perimetry, SAP) taken with the Humphrey Field Analyzer 3 (Carl Zeiss Meditec, Dublin, CA, USA) using the central 24-2 Swedish Interactive Threshold Algorithm strategy (SITA). Mean deviation (MD), pattern standard deviation (PSD), and Glaucoma Staging System 2 (GSS2) classification were registered [4].

The global average thickness (G) of the peripapillary retinal nerve fiber layer (pRNFL) was also registered via Heidelberg Spectralis II OCT (Software Version 6.15, Heidelberg Engineering, Heidelberg, Germany).

The number of different antiglaucoma topical medications applied daily by TMT patients was recorded.

At the end of the visit, the Italian versions of Glaucoma Symptoms Scale (GSS) [19–22] questionnaire and the 25-Item National Eye Institute Visual Functioning Questionnaire (25-NEI-VFQ) [23–25] were administered to each patient's compilation according to the questionnaires' specific compilation guidelines. Each eye was analyzed separately.

The GSS [19–22] questionnaire consists of ten questions related to ten eye complaints that are common in glaucoma patients; they are divided into two groups: six non-visual symptoms (burning, tearing, dryness, itching, irritation, feeling of foreign body) and four visual symptoms (blurred vision, difficulty seeing in daylight, difficulty seeing in darkness, halos around lights). Each symptom is analyzed in terms of presence and annoyance using a scale from 0 to 100 (0 indicates an intense symptom, and 100 corresponds to its absence): the higher the score, the greater the ocular wellbeing. Three scores are finally given: GEN is the total GSS score (mean of the ten subscale scores), SYM is the non-visual symptoms score (mean of the six subscales), and FUNC is the visual symptoms score (mean of the four subscales).

The 25-NEI-VFQ [23–25] consists of 25 main questions and an appendix of 13 additional items grouped in 12 subscales which investigate different fields of the vision-related QoL: general health, general vision, ocular pain, near activities, distance activities, social functioning, mental health, role difficulties, dependency, driving, color vision, and peripheral vision. Patients are required to estimate the fatigue encountered in performing a given daily activity, describing it as absent, small, moderate, severe, or so intense that they can't carry it out. Answers are then converted into a numerical score, then the average for each subscale is calculated going from 0 to 100, where a higher score represents a better QoL.

Statistical Analysis

Group homogeneity was checked via analysis of variance (ANOVA, $p > 0.05$) and proportion tests ($p > 0.05$). Quantitative variables were expressed in terms of mean $\pm$ standard deviations (SD). Regarding both questionnaires' results, the comparison of CP and TB was assessed with the Wilcoxon test, whereas the Kruskal–Wallis test and G-test were required when analyzing CP, TB, and TMT. A p-value < 0.05 was considered statistically significant. Pearson's correlation coefficient (r) was analyzed to study the correlation between QoL and the glaucoma stage (according to GSS2) and between QoL and G value; a corresponding correlation test was used to check the statistical significance.

Statistical analyses were performed using R software 3.6.1 (R Foundation for Statistical Computing, Vienna, Austria).

3. Results

A total of 291 eyes (145 right eyes, 146 left eyes) of 167 Caucasian patients (75 males and 92 females) met the inclusion criteria; the mean age of the study subjects was 77 years (SD, 8 years). Baseline characteristics of the three groups were similar in terms of age and gender according to ANOVA ($p > 0.05$) and proportion tests ($p > 0.05$). Out of 291 included eyes, 92 eyes (31.7%) underwent CP, 56 (19.2%) underwent TB, and 143 (49.1%) were treated with TMT. Regarding TMT patients, a mean number of 1.78 $\pm$ 0.74 different topical anti-hypertensive medications were instilled daily.

Visual field test results are reported in Table 1.

Table 1. Visual field test results in the three different treatment groups.

Parameters	Canaloplasty	Trabeculectomy	Topical Medical Therapy
MD [1]	−13.65 $\pm$ 9.01	−16.88 $\pm$ 8.90	−6.70 $\pm$ 8.21
PSD [2]	8.21 $\pm$ 4.35	8.33 $\pm$ 3.53	4.96 $\pm$ 3.92
GSS2 [3]	3.36 $\pm$ 1.79	3.95 $\pm$ 1.45	1.84 $\pm$ 1.87

[1] Mean Deviation. [2] Pattern Standard Deviation. [3] Glaucoma Staging System 2. Values are reported as mean $\pm$ standard deviation.

The three groups were composed of patients affected by statistically significant different stages of glaucomatous visual field defect according to GSS2 ($p < 0.001$, ANOVA test), as shown in Figure 1. In addition, a statistically significant difference for MD, PSD, and GSS2 between the CP and TB groups was found ($p < 0.001$, ANOVA test).

As regards pRNFL, for the CP group, mean G was 60.51 µm $\pm$ 19 µm, for the TB group, mean G was 58.41 µm $\pm$ 20.2 µm, and for the TMT group, mean G was 75.71 µm $\pm$ 22.5 µm.

The difference among the G values of the three groups was statistically significant ($p < 0.001$, ANOVA test), as shown in Figure 2.

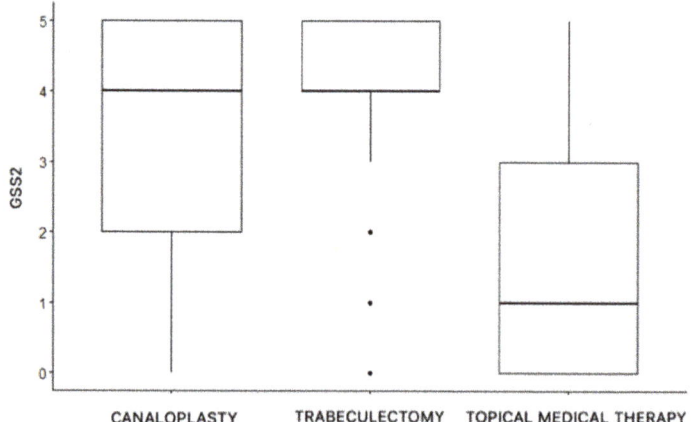

Figure 1. Visual field defect stages according to GSS2 in the three treatments groups.

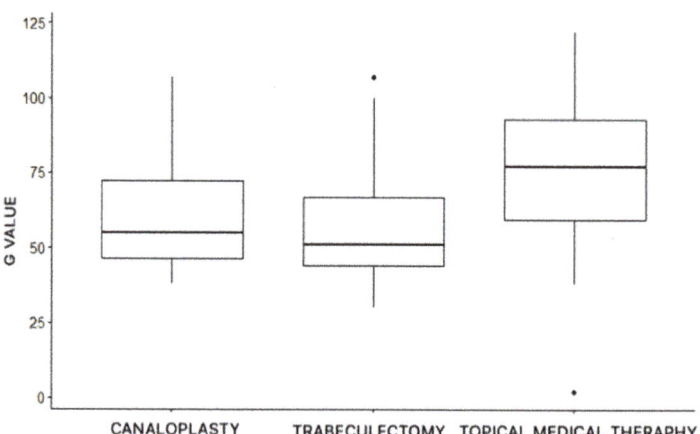

Figure 2. Global average thickness (G value) of the peripapillary retinal nerve fiber layer (pRNFL) in the three treatments groups.

Visual field tests and pRNFL acquisitions images are shown in Figure 3. GSS questionnaire results are reported in Figure 4, Tables 2 and 3.

Table 2. Glaucoma Symptoms Scale (GSS) questionnaire: a comparison between canaloplasty and trabeculectomy through the Wilcoxon test.

Parameters	Canaloplasty	Trabeculectomy	p-Value (Wilcoxon)
GEN [1]	83.3 ± 16.7	80.3 ± 16	0.12
SYM [2]	87.6 ± 15.1	85.2 ± 13.4	0.09
FUNC [3]	76.2 ± 27.9	73.8 ± 26.2	0.36

[1] Total GSS score. [2] Non visual symptoms GSS score. [3] Visual function GSS score. Values are reported as mean ± standard deviation.

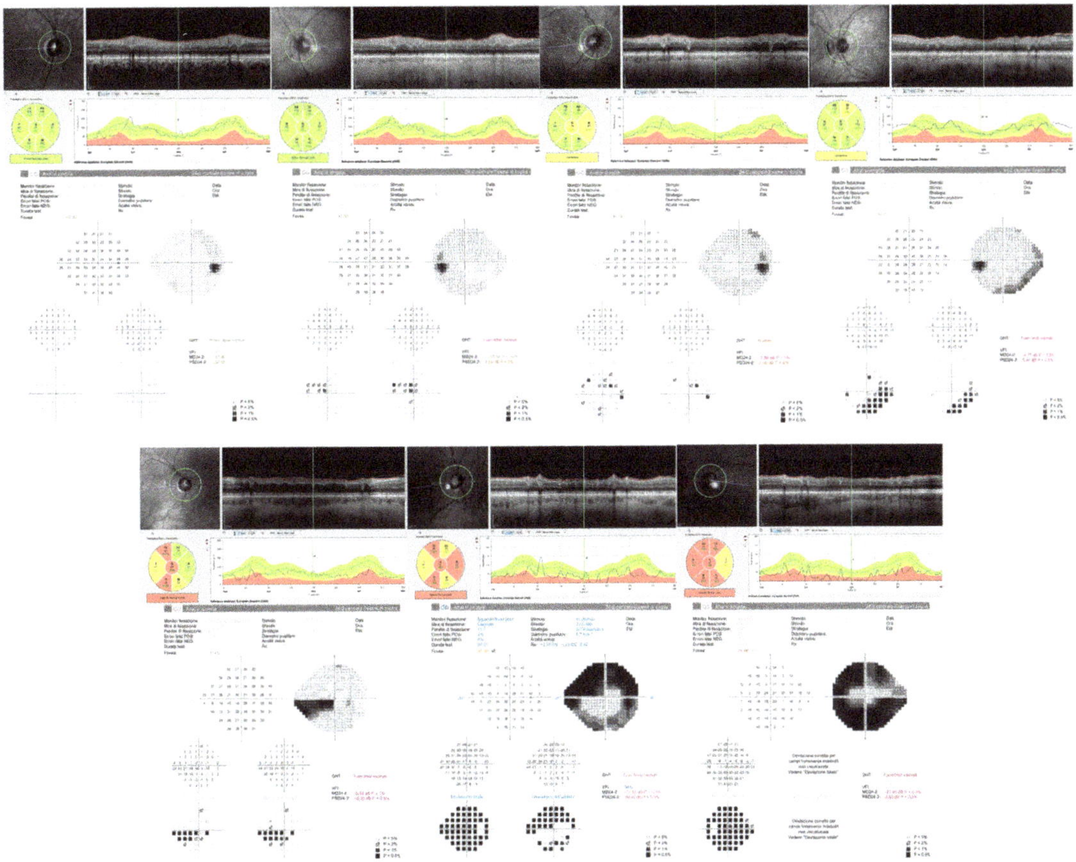

Figure 3. Peripapillary retinal nerve fiber layer and visual fields of patients with different glaucoma stages according to Glaucoma Staging System 2. From left to right, top: stage 0, borderline, 1, 2. From left to right, bottom: stage 3, 4, 5.

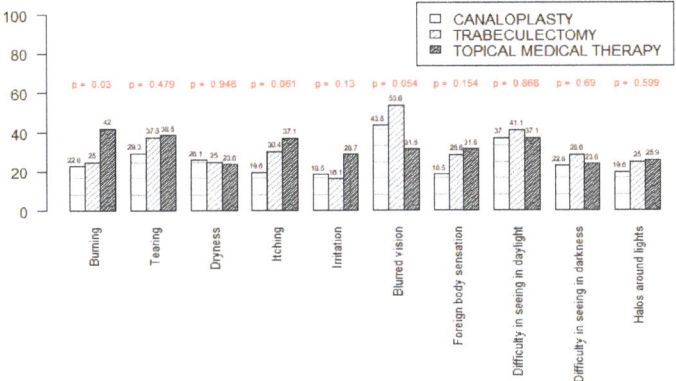

Figure 4. Incidence of the 10 symptoms analyzed by Glaucoma Symptom Scale (GSS) questionnaire in the three treatment groups. *p*-values resulting from the G-test are reported on the top of the columns.

Table 3. Glaucoma Symptoms Scale (GSS) questionnaire: comparison between canaloplasty, trabeculectomy and topical medical therapy through the Kruskal–Wallis test.

Parameters	Canaloplasty	Trabeculectomy	Topical Medical Therapy	p-Value (Kruskal–Wallis)
GEN [1]	83.3 ± 16.7	80.3 ± 16	78.4 ± 20.7	0.18
SYM [2]	87.6 ± 15.1	85.2 ± 13.4	78.8 ± 22.7	**0.006**
FUNC [3]	76.2 ± 27.9	73.8 ± 26.2	78.5 ± 24.5	0.41

[1] Total GSS score. [2] Non visual symptoms GSS score. [3] Visual function GSS score. Values are reported as mean ± standard deviation. Statistically significant results are reported in bold text.

Firstly, the incidence of the 10 symptoms analyzed by the GSS questionnaire in the three treatment groups was analyzed (Figure 3); a statistically significant difference was noted in the incidence of "burning", which was more frequently reported by TMT patients ($p = 0.03$, G test), whereas "blurred vision" was slightly correlated to TB treatment ($p = 0.054$, G test).

Annoyance of symptoms was also studied. Table 2 shows the comparison between CP and TB. CP patients referred a greater QoL: they reported higher (thus better) scores in SYM, FUNC and GEN; however, no statistically significant difference was found (Wilcoxon test).

Table 3 illustrates the comparison among CP, TB, and TMT group; CP patients reported a statistically significant lower annoyance of non-visual symptoms ($p = 0.006$).

The following parameters from the 25-NEI-VFQ were analyzed: general health, general vision, near vision, distance vision, mental health, and peripheral vision. Table 4 shows the comparison between CP and TB patients (Wilcoxon test).

Table 4. General health, general vision, near vision, distance vision, mental health, and peripheral vision parameters of the 25-Item National Eye Institute Visual Functioning Questionnaire (25-NEI-VFQ): comparison between canaloplasty and trabeculectomy through the Wilcoxon test.

Parameters	Canaloplasty	Trabeculectomy	p-Value (Wilcoxon)
General health	68.3 ± 19.5	66 ± 17.1	0.38
General vision	73.2 ± 17.5	63 ± 21	**0.005**
Near vision	86.2 ± 21.9	86.1 ± 25.4	0.54
Distance vision	88.2 ± 18.1	89.3 ± 19.4	0.53
Mental health	78 ± 28.8	81.9 ± 23.3	0.73
Peripheral vision	88 ± 20.8	92 ± 21.2	0.20

Values are reported as mean ± standard deviation. Statistically significant results are reported in bold text.

CP patients reported higher and better scores in general vision than TB patients, and the difference was statistically significant ($p = 0.005$).

The comparison among CP, TB, and the TMT group (Kruskal–Wallis) is reported in Table 5.

Table 5. General health, general vision, near vision, distance vision, mental health and peripheral vision parameters of the 25-Item National Eye Institute Visual Functioning Questionnaire (25-NEI-VFQ): comparison between canaloplasty, trabeculectomy and topical medical therapy through the Kruskal–Wallis test.

Parameters	Canaloplasty	Trabeculectomy	Topical Medical Therapy	p-Value (Kruskal–Wallis)
General health	68.3 ± 19.5	66 ± 171	67.2 ± 20.1	0.67
General vision	73.2 ± 17.5	63 ± 21	68.1 ± 19.2	**0.01**
Near vision	86.2 ± 21.9	86.1 ± 25.4	90.1 ± 19.6	0.29
Distance vision	88.2 ± 18.1	89.3 ± 19.4	91.5 ± 15.2	0.46
Mental health	78 ± 28.8	81.9 ± 23.3	83.8 ± 23.9	0.37
Peripheral vision	88 ± 20.8	92 ± 21.2	93.7 ± 15.8	**0.04**

Values are reported as mean ± standard deviation. Statistically significant results are reported in bold text.

The best results in general vision and peripheral vision were achieved by CP patients, whereas TB patients reported the lowest results; the differences were statistically significant ($p = 0.01$ and $p = 0.04$, respectively).

The Pearson correlation test was performed to assess the presence of a linear correlation between the QoL and functional and anatomical glaucomatous damage. Patients were considered as a single group, regardless of the type of treatment. No statistically significant correlation was found between QoL and the GSS2 stage. A weak positive correlation was found between pRNFL and the following subscales of the GSS questionnaire and the 25-NEI-VFQ: FUNC ($r = 0.213$, $p < 0.001$), general vision ($r = 0.165$, $p = 0.0067$), near activities ($r = 0.244$, $p < 0.001$), distance activities ($r = 0.228$, $p < 0.001$), mental health ($r = 0.192$, $p = 0.0015$), and peripheral vision ($r = 0.27$, $p < 0.001$).

Finally, a linear regression between general vision and MD, PSD, GSS2, and type of surgery was checked. We found a statistically significant regression coefficient ($p = 0.0016$) for type of surgery, with an improvement in the general vision of more than 10.3 points in CP compared to TB group.

4. Discussion

European Glaucoma Society's guidelines state that the aim of glaucoma therapeutic management is the preservation of VF and of a good QoL [10]. According to the guidelines, medical therapy should be the first therapeutic approach. If it fails, surgical treatment is recommended. Currently, the gold standard of surgical therapy is represented by TB [10]. To avoid the above-mentioned complications, CP was developed; this surgical procedure is associated with a lower complication rate and it could represent both an effective and safe therapeutic strategy, which protects the surgeon from the burden of complications and preserves the patient's wellbeing. This was confirmed by Klink et al. [26], who compared the 25-NEI-VFQ results of CP and TB patients, highlighting that VF was considerably better after CP; this kind of surgery was associated with a more preserved ability to read, watch television, see in the dark, and drive, having a lower impact on daily activities. Our study is consistent with this result; we found that CP guarantees a statistically significant better general vision score than TB ($p = 0.005$; Table 4). This is an encouraging outcome, since VF preservation constitutes the therapeutic goal to be achieved. CP does not require the presence of a filtering bleb, avoiding problems associated with it coming in touch with the cornea; this occurrence can cause keratopathy, tear film alterations, and eye surface damage, which can result in a worsening of visual performance [27,28].

In our study, we also evaluated the impact of TMT on QoL and compared it to the two above-mentioned surgical techniques. No available scientific study has provided a contextual comparison of these three therapeutic approaches yet; however, this evaluation could have important implications in clinical practice. Together with IOP reduction, surgery aims to preserve patients' wellbeing and autonomy; it should lead to an improvement in patient QoL, since it virtually reduces the impact of ocular and systemic side effects of TMT, alleviating glaucoma interference in everyday life.

It has already been shown that TB surgery does not fulfill these purposes. In fact, Guedes et al. [29] compared the QoL of TMT patients with those who had undergone surgery (TB, laser iridotomy, and other techniques, but not CP), and those who required mixed therapy. The first group reported significantly better scores on the 25-NEI-VFQ, except for general health and driving, where the differences were not statistically significant. In the CIGTS (The Collaborative Initial Glaucoma Treatment Study) [30], 607 newly diagnosed patients were randomized to TMT or TB surgery and then underwent a 60-month follow-up, during which the impact on QoL of the two different therapies was assessed. One year after surgery, both ocular symptoms and VF were worse in the TB group.

In our study, according to GSS2 results, TMT was associated with the highest incidence of eye burning ($p = 0.03$), whereas blurred vision was more frequent in the TB group ($p = 0.054$). Moreover, CP patients reported the lowest annoyance of non-visual symptoms compared to TB and TMT patients, and the difference was statistically significant ($p = 0.006$).

As far as vision-related QoL is concerned, the 25-NEI-VFQ results show that CP is associated with greater values in the general vision parameter ($p = 0.01$) compared both to the TB group and the TMT group.

It was expected that CP surgery could be associated with a greater QoL than TB. Klink et al. [26] already showed that this minimally invasive and bleb-free procedure is linked to lower eye discomfort and a lower complication rate than TB; moreover, this technique does not require intraoperative and postoperative subconjunctival use of antiproliferative substances, whose application in TB surgery contributes to symptom development. As is known, the postoperative course could be challenging for each surgery; however, after CP, follow-up seems to be easier and most of the patients do not complain about eye discomfort, whereas TB is associated with longer hospitalization and follow-up, a higher chance of a second admission, and more frequent eye examinations (14.5% against 7.5% in canaloplasty) [26–28,31,32].

It was not expected that any surgery could guarantee a significantly better QoL than TMT; interestingly, in our study, CP seemed to achieve this goal. A likely reason for its supremacy can be found in the relationship between eye drops and Ocular Surface Disease (OSD). Pahljina et al. found that a reduction in the number of eye medications following glaucoma surgery (namely, phacoemulsification combined with the Xen gel stent) had a positive impact on patient QoL, according to the GSS questionnaire [33]. OSD affects 15% of healthy people over 65 years of age and 59% of glaucomatous patients; besides aging, one of the most important risk factors for its onset is eye drop instillation and years of treatment [11,34]. The damage is caused both by the active principle and the preservative. Benzalkonium chloride is the most widely used preservative; even at low concentrations, it exerts a toxic effect on the corneal-conjunctival surface, as it accumulates in the eye surface causing cell membrane lysis and altering corneal epithelial and Langerhans cell density; moreover, it determines a poorer tear production and interferes with the integrity of the superficial tear lipid layer, decreasing its stability, as demonstrated by the reduction in the break-up time [5,35].

Rossi et al. analyzed the relation between OSD and QoL in glaucoma patients receiving eye drops containing benzalkonium chloride through the 25-NEI-VFQ and the GSS questionnaires. Patients with OSD reached low mean total scores; the same results were obtained when dry eye syndrome was valued [11,35,36]. These conditions reduce visual performance and can limit daily activities such as reading, working on the computer, or driving. According to Van Gestel et al. [37], OSD seems to have a greater impact on QoL than the disease progression [36]; however, preservation of central and near vision, mobility, and daily activities is considered more important than the absence of eye discomfort, even by patients.

As regards peripheral vision, the TMT group gained the highest scores, and the difference turned out to be statistically significant ($p = 0.04$); this could be expected, since glaucoma visual field damage is typically centripetal, and this group was characterized by earlier GSS2 stages.

The supremacy of CP over TMT represents an interesting finding, considering that CP patients were affected by more advanced stages of anatomical and functional damage. Previous studies reported a correlation between the 25-NEI-VFQ results and visual field deterioration [7,20,38]. In our study, we found no correlation between the QoL and GSS2. Patients' wellbeing seemed not to depend just on the progression of the perimetric defect; it represents a wider concept, influenced by numerous variables, which should be considered when evaluating the effectiveness of a given treatment. On the other hand, a linear positive correlation between QoL and pRNLF emerged. The relationship between anatomical changes and QoL is still not clear [39]. In a longitudinal study, Gracitelli et al. [40] already described how progressive thinning of RNFL was associated with a decrease in QoL over time. They reported that each 1-µm-per-year reduction in RNFL thickness corresponded to a modification in the 25-NEI-VFQ scores of 1.1 units per year; the association was confirmed even after accounting for visual field loss over time. This could partially explain why we found an anatomical correlation but not a functional one. Structural assessment seems to provide additional information for predicting change in QoL beyond what SAP can reveal; according to authors, there may be adjunctive visual changes that are relevant to QoL but cannot be fully captured by SAP, such as motion perception.

We also performed a correlation between the GSS questionnaire results and pRNLF; it is interesting to notice that a positive correlation was found for the visual symptoms (FUNC) subscale but not for the non-visual symptoms (SYM) subscale. Floriani et al. reported similar results when correlating GSS questionnaire's results and GSS2 stages [7]. In our study, the impact of ocular disturbances (such as burning) on QoL shows no correlation with optic neuropathy, supporting our hypothesis that the type of treatment may have a role in determining patients' wellbeing.

Limitations of the present study are its retrospective design and the small sample size. Moreover, as known, QoL can be affected by additional comorbidities, both ocular and systemic; nevertheless, since the three groups were homogeneous by sex and age, it is reasonable to assume that such pathologies also had a similar distribution. Future studies should aim to include a larger number of patients, have a prospective design, and a longer follow-up period.

5. Conclusions

CP seems to provide a better QoL when compared to both TB and TMT, guaranteeing better general vision, fewer symptoms, and a lower rate of complications. pRNFL thinning correlates with VR-QoL and seems to provide additional information on its changing besides what visual field test can reveal. However, local symptoms seem not to depend only on the structural damage, and the impact of treatment may be relevant. According to our findings, CP helps to combine IOP control with the need to ensure the patient's wellbeing. Undergoing this kind of surgery, the patient will not have to instill topical drugs, avoiding their side effects; on the other hand, they will not face bleb-related ocular disorders, as in the case of TB. After a few weeks, the patient will be free from ocular discomfort. These findings suggest that CP could represent a valid therapeutic alternative in patients who poorly adhere to medical instruction or do not tolerate TMT; the lower rate of complications suggests it should be proposed more confidently even to younger patients, who will also benefit from the more delayed follow-ups.

Author Contributions: Conceptualization, M.R.P.; methodology, M.R.P. and L.E.; software, validation, formal analysis, investigation, and resources, M.R.P., S.M., R.A., L.E., T.A., L.B., G.C. and D.T.; data curation, M.R.P. and S.M.; writing—original draft preparation, S.M. and R.A.; writing—review and editing, M.R.P. and S.M.; visualization, supervision, M.R.P., S.M., R.A., L.E., T.A., L.B., G.C. and D.T.; project administration, M.R.P. and D.T. All authors have read and agreed to the published version of the manuscript.

Funding: This research received no external funding.

Institutional Review Board Statement: The study was conducted in accordance with the Declaration of Helsinki, and approved by the Institutional Review Board of the University of Trieste (No. 108/2020, 19 October 2020).

Informed Consent Statement: Informed consent was obtained from all subjects involved in the study.

Data Availability Statement: Data are available on reasonable request by the corresponding author.

Conflicts of Interest: The authors declare no conflict of interest.

References

1. Hu, C.X.; Zangalli, C.; Hsieh, M.; Gupta, L.; Williams, A.L.; Richman, J.; Spaeth, G.L. What do patients with glaucoma see? Visual symptoms reported by patients with glaucoma. *Am. J. Med. Sci.* **2014**, *348*, 403–409. [CrossRef] [PubMed]
2. Bierings, R.A.J.M.; Kuiper, M.; Van Berkel, C.M.; Overkempe, T.; Jansonius, N.M. Foveal light and dark adaptation in patients with glaucoma and healthy subjects: A case-control study. *PLoS ONE* **2018**, *13*, e0193663. [CrossRef] [PubMed]

3. Bierings, R.A.J.M.; van Sonderen, F.L.P.; Jansonius, N.M. Visual complaints of patients with glaucoma and controls under optimal and extreme luminance conditions. *Acta Ophthalmol.* **2018**, *96*, 288–294. [CrossRef]
4. Riva, I.; Legramandi, L.; Rulli, E.; Konstas, A.G.; Katsanos, A.; Oddone, F.; Weinreb, R.N.; Quaranta, L.; Varano, L.; Carchedi, T.; et al. Vision-related quality of life and symptom perception change over time in newly-diagnosed primary open angle glaucoma patients. *Sci. Rep.* **2019**, *9*, 6735. [CrossRef] [PubMed]
5. Quaranta, L.; Riva, I.; Gerardi, C.; Oddone, F.; Floriano, I.; Konstas, A.G.P. Quality of Life in Glaucoma: A Review of the Literature. *Adv. Ther.* **2016**, *33*, 959–981. [CrossRef] [PubMed]
6. Mangione, C.M.; Berry, S.; Spritzer, K.; Janz, N.K.; Klein, R.; Owsley, C.; Lee, P.P. Identifying the Content Area for the 51-Item National Eye Institute Visual Function Questionnaire. *Arch. Ophthalmol.* **1998**, *116*, 227–233. [CrossRef]
7. Floriani, I.; Quaranta, L.; Rulli, E.; Katsanos, A.; Varano, L.; Frezzotti, P.; Rossi, G.C.M.; Carmassi, L.; Rolle, T.; Ratiglia, R.; et al. Health-related quality of life in patients with primary open-angle glaucoma. An Italian multicentre observational study. *Acta Ophthalmol.* **2016**, *94*, e278–e286. [CrossRef]
8. Khorrami-nejad, M.; Sarabandi, A.; Akbari, M.-R.; Askarizadeh, F. The Impact of Visual Impairment on Quality of Life. *Med. Hypothesis Discov. Innov. Ophthalmol.* **2016**, *5*, 96. Available online: https://www.ncbi.nlm.nih.gov/pmc/articles/PMC5347211/pdf/mehdiophth-5-096.pdf (accessed on 10 July 2022).
9. Wu, N.; Kong, X.; Gao, J.; Sun, X. Vision-related Quality of Life in Glaucoma Patients and its Correlations with Psychological Disturbances and Visual Function Indices. *J. Glaucoma* **2019**, *28*, 207–215. [CrossRef]
10. European Glaucoma Society. *Terminology and Guidelines for Glaucoma*; PubliComm: Savona, Italy, 2014; ISBN 9788898320059.
11. Rossi, G.C.M.; Pasinetti, G.M.; Scudeller, L.; Bianchi, P.E. Ocular surface disease and glaucoma: How to evaluate impact on quality of life. *J. Ocul. Pharmacol. Ther.* **2013**, *29*, 390–394. [CrossRef]
12. Miguel, A.I.M.; Fonseca, C.; Oliveira, N.; Henriques, F.; Silva, J.F. Difficulties of daily tasks in advanced glaucoma patients—A videotaped evaluation. *Rev. Bras. Oftalmol.* **2015**, *74*, 164–170. [CrossRef]
13. Hugues, F.C.; Le Jeunne, C. Systemic and Local Tolerability of Ophthalmic Drug Formulations: An Update. *Drug Saf.* **1993**, *8*, 365–380. [CrossRef] [PubMed]
14. Zhang, B.; Kang, J.; Chen, X. A System Review and Meta-Analysis of Canaloplasty Outcomes in Glaucoma Treatment in Comparison with Trabeculectomy. *J. Ophthalmol.* **2017**, *2017*, 2723761. [CrossRef] [PubMed]
15. Liu, H.; Zhang, H.; Li, Y.; Yu, H. Safety and efficacy of canaloplasty versus trabeculectomy in treatment of glaucoma. *Oncotarget* **2017**, *8*, 44811–44818. [CrossRef] [PubMed]
16. Lin, Z.J.; Xu, S.; Huang, S.Y.; Zhang, X.B.; Zhong, Y.S. Comparison of canaloplasty and trabeculectomy for open angle glaucoma: A meta-analysis. *Int. J. Ophthalmol.* **2016**, *9*, 1814–1819. [CrossRef]
17. Riva, I.; Brusini, P.; Oddone, F.; Michelessi, M.; Weinreb, R.N.; Quaranta, L. Canaloplasty in the Treatment of Open-Angle Glaucoma: A Review of Patient Selection and Outcomes. *Adv. Ther.* **2019**, *36*, 31–43. [CrossRef]
18. Ayyala, R.S.; Chaudhry, A.L.; Okogbaa, C.B.; Zurakowski, D. Comparison of Surgical Outcomes Between Canaloplasty and Trabeculectomy at 12 Months' Follow-Up. *Ophthalmology* **2011**, *118*, 2427–2433. [CrossRef]
19. Lee, B.L.; Gutierrez, P.; Gordon, M.; Wilson, M.R.; Cioffi, G.A.; Ritch, R.; Sherwood, M.; Mangione, C.M.; Stein, J. The Glaucoma Symptom Scale. *Arch. Ophthalmol.* **1998**, *116*, 861–866. [CrossRef]
20. Rulli, E.; Quaranta, L.; Riva, I.; Poli, D.; Hollander, L.; Galli, F.; Katsanos, A.; Oddone, F.; Torri, V.; Weinreb, R.N.; et al. Visual field loss and vision-related quality of life in the Italian Primary Open Angle Glaucoma Study. *Sci. Rep.* **2018**, *8*, 619. [CrossRef]
21. Vercellin Verticchio, A.C.; Vento, M.; Pasinetti, G.M.; Raimondi, M.; Lanteri, S.; Lombardo, S.; Rossi, G.C.M. Traduzione, validazione e affidabilità della versione italiana del questionario Glaucoma Symptom Scale. *Boll. Soc. Med. Chir. Pavia* **2012**, *125*, 483–495. [CrossRef]
22. Kass, M.A. The ocular hypertension treatment study. *J. Glaucoma* **1994**, *3*, 97–100. [CrossRef] [PubMed]
23. Wang, Y.; Alnwisi, S.; Ke, M. The impact of mild, moderate, and severe visual field loss in glaucoma on patients' quality of life measured via the Glaucoma Quality of Life-15 Questionnaire. *Medicine* **2017**, *96*, e8019. [CrossRef] [PubMed]
24. Mangione, C.M.; Lee, P.P.; Pitts, J.; Gutierrez, P.; Berry, S.; Hays, R.D. Psychometric properties of the National Eye Institute Visual Function Questionnaire (NEI-VFQ). *Arch. Ophthalmol.* **1998**, *116*, 1496–1504. [CrossRef]
25. Rossi, G.C.M.; Milano, G.; Tinelli, C. The Italian version of the 25-item National Eye Institute Visual Function Questionnaire: Translation, validity, and reliability. *J. Glaucoma* **2003**, *12*, 213–220. [CrossRef]
26. Klink, T.; Sauer, J.; Körber, N.J.; Grehn, F.; Much, M.M.; Thederan, L.; Matlach, J.; Salgado, J.P. Quality of life following glaucoma surgery: Canaloplasty versus trabeculectomy. *Clin. Ophthalmol.* **2014**, *9*, 7–16. [CrossRef]
27. Vijaya, L.; Manish, P.; Shantha, B. Management of complications in glaucoma surgery. *Indian J. Ophthalmol.* **2011**, *59* (Suppl. S1), S131–S140. [CrossRef] [PubMed]
28. Zarbin, M.; Hersh, P.; Haynes, W.L.; Alward, W.L.M. Control of Intraocular Pressure After Trabeculectomy. *Surv. Ophthalmol.* **1999**, *43*, 345–355.
29. Guedes, R.A.P.; Guedes, V.M.P.; Freitas, S.M.; Chaoubah, A. Quality of life of glaucoma patients under medical therapy with different prostaglandins. *Clin. Ophthalmol.* **2012**, *6*, 1749–1753. [CrossRef] [PubMed]
30. Janz, N.K.; Wren, P.A.; Lichter, P.R.; Musch, D.C.; Gillespie, B.W.; Guire, K.E.; Mills, R.P.; CIGTS Study Group. The collaborative initial glaucoma treatment study: Interim quality of life findings after initial medical or surgical treatment of glaucoma. *Ophthalmology* **2001**, *108*, 1954–1965. [CrossRef]

31. Lewis, R.A.; von Wolff, K.; Tetz, M.; Korber, N.; Kearney, J.R.; Shingleton, B.; Samuelson, T.W. Canaloplasty: Circumferential viscodilation and tensioning of Schlemm's canal using a flexible microcatheter for the treatment of open-angle glaucoma in adults. Interim clinical study analysis. *J. Cataract Refract. Surg.* **2007**, *33*, 1217–1226. [CrossRef]
32. Taube, A.B.; Niemelä, P.; Alm, A. Trabeculectomy with an active postoperative regimen: Results and resource utilization. *Acta Ophthalmol.* **2009**, *87*, 524–528. [CrossRef] [PubMed]
33. Pahljina, C.; Sarny, S.; Hoeflechner, L.; Falb, T.; Schliessleder, G.; Lindner, M.; Ivastinovic, D.; Mansouri, K.; Lindner, E. Glaucoma Medication and Quality of Life after Phacoemulsification Combined with a Xen Gel Stent. *J. Clin. Med.* **2022**, *11*, 3450. [CrossRef] [PubMed]
34. Moss, S.E.; Klein, R.; Klein, B.E.K. Prevalance of and risk factors for dry eye syndrome. *Arch. Ophthalmol.* **2000**, *118*, 1264–1268. [CrossRef] [PubMed]
35. Kovačević, S.; Čanović, S.; Didović Pavičić, A.; Kolega, M.Š.; Bašić, J.K. Ocular surface changes in glaucoma patients related to topical medications. *Coll. Antropol.* **2015**, *39*, 47–49.
36. Rossi, G.C.M.; Tinelli, C.; Pasinetti, G.M.; Milano, G.; Bianchi, P.E. Dry eye syndrome-related quality of life in glaucoma patients. *Eur. J. Ophthalmol.* **2009**, *19*, 572–579. [CrossRef]
37. Van Gestel, A.; Webers, C.A.B.; Beckers, H.J.M.; Van Dongen, M.C.J.M.; Severens, J.L.; Hendrikse, F.; Schouten, J.S.A.G. The relationship between visual field loss in glaucoma and health-related quality-of-life. *Eye* **2010**, *24*, 1759–1769. [CrossRef]
38. Labiris, G.; Katsanos, A.; Fanariotis, M.; Zacharaki, F.; Chatzoulis, D.; Kozobolis, V.P. Vision-specific quality of life in Greek glaucoma patients. *J. Glaucoma* **2010**, *19*, 39–43. [CrossRef]
39. Hirneiß, C.; Reznicek, L.; Vogel, M.; Pesudovs, K. The impact of structural and functional parameters in glaucoma patients on patient-reported visual functioning. *PLoS ONE* **2013**, *8*, e80757. [CrossRef]
40. Gracitelli, C.P.; Abe, R.Y.; Tatham, A.J.; Rosen, P.N.; Zangwill, L.M.; Boer, E.R.; Weinreb, R.N.; Medeiros, F.A. Association between progressive retinal nerve fiber layer loss and longitudinal change in quality of life in glaucoma. *JAMA Ophthalmol.* **2015**, *133*, 384–390. [CrossRef]

Article
Optical Coherence Tomography Analysis of Retinal Layers in Celiac Disease

Livio Vitiello [1], Maddalena De Bernardo [1,*], Luca Erra [1], Federico Della Rocca [2], Nicola Rosa [1] and Carolina Ciacci [2]

1. Eye Unit, Department of Medicine, Surgery and Dentistry, "Scuola Medica Salernitana", University of Salerno, 84081 Salerno, Italy
2. Celiac Centre at University Hospital San Giovanni Di Dio e Ruggi d'Aragona, University of Salerno, 84084 Salerno, Italy
* Correspondence: mdebernardo@unisa.it

Abstract: Celiac disease is an immune-mediated, chronic, inflammatory, and systemic illness which could affect the eye. The aim of this study is to look for possible signs of retinal involvement in celiac disease that could be utilized as biomarkers for this disease. Sixty-six patients with celiac disease and sixty-six sex-matched healthy subjects were enrolled in this observational case–control study. A comprehensive ophthalmological evaluation, axial length measurements, and SD-OCT evaluation were performed. The thickness of the retinal layers at the circle centered on the fovea (1 mm in diameter) and the average of the foveal and parafoveal zones at 2 and 3 mm in diameter were evaluated, together with retinal volume and the peripapillary retinal nerve fiber layer (RNFL). Concerning the thicknesses of the retinal layers in each analyzed region, no statistically significant differences were found. The same results were obtained for the total volume. Regarding peripapillary RNFL, the celiac patients showed slightly thicker values than the healthy controls, except for temporal and nasal-inferior quadrants, with no statistically significant differences. All the analyzed parameters were similar for the celiac patients and the healthy individuals. This could be related either to the non-involvement of the retinal layers in celiac disease pathophysiology or to the gluten-free diet effect.

Keywords: celiac disease; OCT; optical coherence tomography; retinal layers; RNFL

1. Introduction

Celiac disease is an immune-mediated, chronic, inflammatory, and systemic illness [1] characterized by the formation of autoantibodies against tissue transglutaminase, which are triggered by gluten and gluten-like proteins in genetically susceptible subjects [2].

Classic celiac disease presents malabsorption, failure to thrive, and diarrhea. At the same time, more subtle presentations such as latent, potential, oligosymptomatic, and extraintestinal signs related to otologic, dental, neurological, dermatological, and musculoskeletal symptoms may be less prevalent [3]. However, individuals are in danger of long-term complications if undetected extraintestinal manifestations are not addressed [4,5].

Among these extraintestinal findings, ocular manifestations due to celiac disease are of great concern because of the direct effect of visual function and ocular comfort on the quality of life [6,7].

The presence of circulating immune complexes or autoantibodies in ocular tissues, cross-reactivity of cell antigenic epitopes, vitamin deficiencies, and immunogenetic factors might all play a role in ocular involvement, especially for all the vascularized components of the eye [6].

In fact, the choroid of celiac patients appears thicker than healthy controls [8,9]. In particular, De Bernardo et al. [9] not only confirmed a thicker choroid in celiac patients [8], but analyzing the choroidal vascularity index in these patients, found no statistical differences between celiac patients and healthy controls. However, celiac patients showed all the choroidal areas to be larger in a significant way than the healthy group. Thus, De Bernardo et al. supposed a proportional increase in both the vascular and stromal components, that may be linked to the inflammatory and autoimmune responses related to celiac disease pathophysiology [9]. On the other hand, anterior eye segment changes due to celiac disease are still unclear [10–12].

To the best of our knowledge, no studies have been published examining all the retinal layers concerning retinal involvement in celiac disease. Only a few studies evaluated the peripapillary retinal nerve fiber layer (RNFL), showing no consensus in children and adults [11–14]. In addition, one study also evaluated the ganglion cell complex (GCC) in a pediatric population, finding no statistical difference between celiac patients and healthy controls [14].

For these reasons, together with the disease's autoimmune and inflammatory nature and the presence of the superficial and deep capillary plexuses among the retinal layers, this study aims to look for possible signs of retinal involvement, utilizing spectral-domain optical coherence tomography (SD-OCT), that could be utilized as biomarkers for this disease.

2. Materials and Methods

2.1. Patient Selection

Adult subjects with a diagnosis of celiac disease, evaluated at the Celiac Disease Center at the Department of Medicine, Surgery, and Dentistry of the University of Salerno between September 2019 and March 2020, and a control group of sex-matched healthy subjects were included in this observational case–control study.

Diagnosis of celiac disease was confirmed by intestinal biopsy and serology, regardless of the time of diagnosis. Following the diagnosis, all the celiac patients were placed on a gluten-free diet. Regarding control subjects, they had at least one negative-specific serology for celiac disease and no diagnosis of any gastrointestinal diseases.

Subjects younger than 18 years of age or with systemic and ocular diseases, or patients who underwent other ophthalmic surgical procedures which could affect the eye [15–18], were excluded from this study.

According to the Declaration of Helsinki's ethical principles, all participants were informed about the study's purpose and written informed consent was acquired. Institutional Review Board approval was also obtained from the ComEtico Campania Sud (CECS), prot. n°16544.

2.2. Clinical Examination and OCT Analysis

A comprehensive ophthalmological evaluation, including clinical history to identify possible exclusion criteria, slit-lamp examination, Snellen best-corrected visual acuity, axial length (AL) measurements with IOLMaster (Carl Zeiss Meditec AG, Jena, Germany, version 5.4.4.0006), and SD-OCT evaluation (Spectralis; Heidelberg Engineering; Heidelberg, Germany, version 6.0), was performed.

All participants were examined between 2:00 p.m. and 3:00 p.m., without pupil dilation. For each participant, only the right eye was evaluated [19].

A horizontal 30° volume OCT B-scan centered on the fovea was obtained for all examined eyes. Using the device's built-in software (Heidelberg Eye Explorer HEYEX; Heidelberg Engineering), the segmentation of the retinal layers was obtained.

Poor-quality images with a signal-to-noise score lower than 20 decibels were excluded. To study the 10 retinal layers, eleven optical interfaces were obtained (Figure 1) [20].

In addition, utilizing the standard Early Treatment Diabetic Retinopathy Study (ETDRS) grid, the thickness of the retinal layers at the circle centered on the fovea (1 mm in diameter), the average of the 5 foveal and parafoveal zones (2 mm in diameter), and the average of the 9 foveal and parafoveal zones (3 mm in diameter) were evaluated (Figure 2).

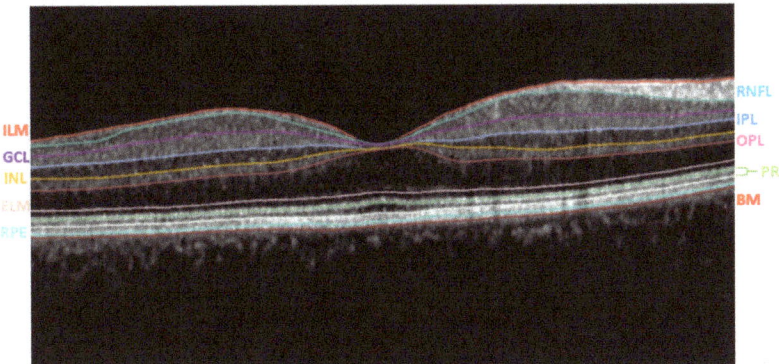

Figure 1. Segmentation of the retinal layers using the instrument's automatic algorithm. ILM: internal limiting membrane; RNFL: retinal nerve fiber layer; GCL: ganglion cell layer; IPL: inner plexiform layer; INL: inner nuclear layer; OPL: outer plexiform layer; ELM: external limiting membrane; PR: photoreceptor layers; RPE: retinal pigment epithelium; BM: Bruch's membrane.

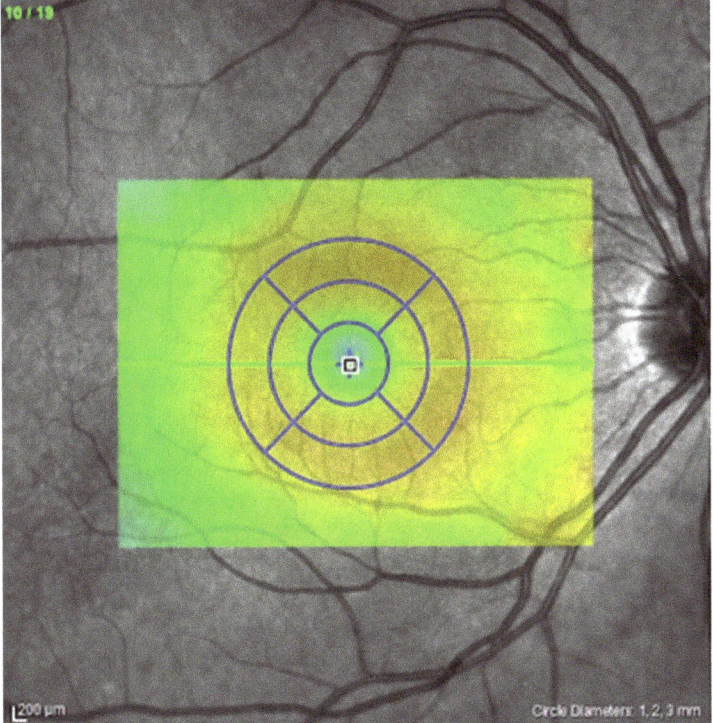

Figure 2. Early Treatment Diabetic Retinopathy Study grid utilized for the retinal analysis.

For all the analyzed regions (1, 2, and 3 mm diameter), the values of the total thickness (total retina), photoreceptor (PHR) layer, retinal pigment epithelium (RPE), outer nuclear layer (ONL), outer plexiform layer (OPL), the inner retinal layer (IRL), and the GCC thickness were collected. IRL includes the sum of RNFL, GCL, IPL, and the inner nuclear layer (INL), while GCC is composed of RNFL, GCL, and IPL. However, the thickness value for all these layers was also evaluated individually in each studied region of the ETDRS grid.

Moreover, the device's built-in software automatically calculated the total volume at 3 mm diameter for each retinal layer.

Concerning peripapillary RNFL, the optic nerve head protocol of the device generates an RNFL thickness map from which RNFL thickness is measured along a circle 3.45 mm in diameter centered on the optic disc. The average RNFL thickness of the seven quadrants (global average, temporal, temporal-superior, nasal-superior, nasal, nasal-inferior, and temporal-inferior) was measured for all patients.

2.3. Statistical Analysis

All data were analyzed with GraphPad Prism 8 (GraphPad Software, LLC, version 8.4.3). Kolmogorov–Smirnov test was performed to assess normal distribution ($p > 0.05$) for all data.

To compare the different parameters of the two groups, the two-tailed Mann–Whitney U test for not normal-distributed data and the two-tailed independent samples Student t-test for normal-distributed data were used. Furthermore, the correlation between the years of gluten-free diet adherence and the total retinal thickness in each analyzed region was also evaluated using the Spearman correlation test. p values less than 0.05 were considered statistically significant.

The sample size was determined by maximizing the statistical power. The analysis was performed using G*Power software (version 3.1.9.4) [21]. A difference between two independent means (two groups) was computed. Input data were the following: α was set at 0.05; 1-β was set at 0.81; allocation ratio N2/N1 was set at 1; and the effect size was set as a medium at around 0.5. Results were the following: non-centrality parameter δ = 2.872; critical t = 1.978; Df = 130; sample size group 1 = 66; sample size group 2 = 66; actual power = 0.814; and total sample size = 132.

3. Results

Sixty-six patients with celiac disease (nineteen males) and sixty-six sex-matched healthy subjects were enrolled. The mean disease duration of the celiac patients was 9.1 ± 8.8 years (range: 0–41 years). None of the celiac patients included in this study presented previous ocular complications due to celiac disease.

The mean age of the celiac patients was 40.3 ± 11.6 years (range: 18–66 years), while the mean age of the healthy subjects was 39.9 ± 14.2 (range: 23–69 years), with no statistically significant difference between the two groups ($p = 0.75$).

The mean AL of the celiac patients was 23.6 ± 1.0 mm (range: 21.7–26.1 mm), while the mean AL of the healthy subjects was 23.9 ± 1.2 mm (range: 20.7–27.5 mm), with no statistically significant difference between the two groups ($p = 0.15$).

Concerning the thicknesses of the retinal layers at each analyzed region of the ETDRS grid, no statistically significant differences were found between the celiac patients and the healthy subjects, as shown in Tables 1–3. However, celiac patients showed slightly thicker retinal layers than healthy subjects, except for INL at 1 mm diameter (Table 1); ONL, INL, and GCL at 2 mm diameter (Table 2); and ONL, GCL, RNFL, and GCC at 3 mm diameter (Table 3).

By comparing the total volume, no statistically significant differences were found as well, as summarized in Table 4.

Regarding peripapillary RNFL, the celiac patients showed slightly thicker values than the healthy controls, except for temporal and nasal-inferior quadrants. Nonetheless, no statistically significant difference for these parameters was found, as shown in Table 5.

Considering the correlation between the years of gluten-free diet adherence and the total retinal thickness, no statistically significant correlation was found at 1 mm ($p = 0.07$; r = −0.23), at 2 mm ($p = 0.15$; r = −0.18), and at 3 mm ($p = 0.53$; r = −0.08).

Table 1. Comparison of average retinal layer thicknesses (μm) between celiac patients and healthy subjects at 1 mm diameter of ETDRS grid on OCT.

	Celiac Patients 19 Males–47 Females		Healthy Controls 19 Males–47 Females		p-Value
	Mean ± SD (Range)	Median (IQ Range)	Mean ± SD (Range)	Median (IQ Range)	
PHR (μm)	88.2 ± 3.3 (82.0–99.0)	88.0 (86.0–90.0)	87.9 ± 3.4 (81.0–95.0)	87.0 (85.8–90.3)	[a] 0.67
IRL (μm)	182.6 ± 17.7 (148.0–221.0)	181.5 (171.8–196.0)	180.7 ± 19.8 (137.0–237.0)	179.0 (167.0–195.0)	[b] 0.57
RPE (μm)	16.1 ± 1.5 (13.0–19.0)	16.0 (15.0–17.0)	15.9 ± 1.8 (12.0–19.0)	16.0 (15.0–17.0)	[a] 0.72
ONL (μm)	92.7 ± 10.2 (65.0–117.0)	92.5 (87.0–100.3)	92.2 ± 9.9 (64.0–115.0)	92.0 (86.8–99.0)	[b] 0.78
OPL (μm)	26.2 ± 5.2 (17.0–41.0)	26.0 (22.0–29.0)	25.6 ± 5.8 (16.0–43.0)	25.0 (21.8–29.0)	[a] 0.55
INL (μm)	18.3 ± 5.1 (9.0–34.0)	18.0 (14.0–21.0)	19.1 ± 5.6 (11.0–37.0)	19.0 (14.8–23.0)	[a] 0.51
IPL (μm)	20.3 ± 3.6 (13.0–29.0)	20.0 (17.0–23.0)	19.5 ± 3.4 (13.0–31.0)	19.0 (17.0–22.0)	[a] 0.39
GCL (μm)	14.6 ± 4.3 (8.0–25.0)	14.0 (12.0–17.0)	13.9 ± 3.9 (7.0–30.0)	13.0 (11.8–16.0)	[a] 0.40
RNFL (μm)	12.2 ± 2.0 (7.0–17.0)	12.0 (11.0–14.0)	11.9 ± 2.4 (7.0–19.0)	12.0 (10.0–13.0)	[a] 0.49
GCC (μm)	46.8 ± 9.3 (28.0–71.0)	46.0 (40.0–53.3)	45.3 ± 9.0 (27.0–77.0)	44.5 (40.0–50.3)	[b] 0.37
TOTAL RETINA (μm)	270.8 ± 18.2 (235.0–308.0)	270.0 (257.5–284.3)	268.6 ± 20.2 (228.0–328.0)	266.0 (254.5–283.3)	[b] 0.52

[a] Mann Whitney U test; [b] Student t-test unpaired. SD: Standard Deviation; IQ: Interquartile; PHR: Photoreceptors; IRL: Inner Retinal Layer; RPE: Retinal Pigment Epithelium; ONL: Outer Nuclear Layer; OPL: Outer Plexiform Layer; INL: Inner Nuclear Layer; IPL: Inner Plexiform Layer; GCL: Ganglion Cell Layer; RNFL: Retinal Nerve Fiber Layer; GCC: Ganglion Cell Complex.

Table 2. Comparison of average retinal layer thicknesses (μm) between celiac patients and healthy subjects at 2 mm diameter of ETDRS grid on OCT.

	Celiac Patients 19 Males–47 Females		Healthy Controls 19 Males–47 Females		p-Value
	Mean ± SD (Range)	Median (IQ Range)	Mean ± SD (Range)	Median (IQ Range)	
PHR (μm)	84.0 ± 3.4 (77.6–95.6)	83.8 (81.8–85.8)	83.6 ± 2.8 (77.4–89.6)	83.8 (81.8–85.8)	[a] 0.48
IRL (μm)	236.2 ± 13.2 (214.2–272.2)	234.4 (226.6–245.6)	235.3 ± 16.5 (193.8–267.6)	234.8 (223.0–250.6)	[a] 0.72
RPE (μm)	15.6 ± 1.5 (12.6–19.8)	15.6 (14.8–16.8)	15.5 ± 1.5 (11.8–18.8)	15.4 (14.2–16.6)	[a] 0.24
ONL (μm)	76.9 ± 9.7 (59.0–103.0)	75.2 (70.9–84.3)	77.0 ± 9.5 (55.0–100.0)	77.7 (70.6–84.4)	[b] 0.79
OPL (μm)	34.6 ± 5.3 (24.8–48.6)	33.9 (31.2–38.5)	33.4 ± 5.6 (24.8–46.0)	31.9 (29.3–37.8)	[b] 0.12
INL (μm)	34.1 ± 4.0 (24.8–44.8)	33.5 (31.4–37.3)	34.5 ± 4.1 (27.8–44.2)	34.4 (30.8–37.4)	[a] 0.61
IPL (μm)	35.7 ± 3.3 (29.2–42.8)	36.2 (34.2–37.9)	35.5 ± 3.7 (27.4–43.6)	35.2 (32.8–38.6)	[a] 0.76
GCL (μm)	39.3 ± 5.2 (27.8–51.4)	39.4 (35.3–43.5)	39.4 ± 5.2 (28.8–50.2)	39.1 (35.6–43.2)	[a] 0.97
RNFL (μm)	16.0 ± 0.9 (13.6–18.6)	15.8 (15.4–16.6)	15.9 ± 1.2 (13.6–20.0)	15.6 (15.0–16.6)	[b] 0.50
GCC (μm)	91.0 ± 8.5 (74.4–112.5)	91.7 (84.9–97.1)	90.8 ± 9.3 (72.2–110.2)	90.2 (84.3–97.6)	[a] 0.90
TOTAL RETINA (μm)	320.3 ± 14.6 (298.4–358.6)	318.9 (308.2–330.9)	318.9 ± 17.0 (272.0–354.8)	318.4 (307.9–329.9)	[a] 0.62

[a] Student t-test unpaired; [b] Mann Whitney U test. SD: Standard Deviation; IQ: Interquartile; PHR: Photoreceptors; IRL: Inner Retinal Layer; RPE: Retinal Pigment Epithelium; ONL: Outer Nuclear Layer; OPL: Outer Plexiform Layer; INL: Inner Nuclear Layer; IPL: Inner Plexiform Layer; GCL: Ganglion Cell Layer; RNFL: Retinal Nerve Fiber Layer; GCC: Ganglion Cell Complex.

Table 3. Comparison of average retinal layer thicknesses (μm) between celiac patients and healthy subjects at 3 mm diameter of ETDRS grid on OCT.

	Celiac Patients 19 Males–47 Females		Healthy Controls 19 Males–47 Females		p-Value
	Mean ± SD (Range)	Median (IQ Range)	Mean ± SD (Range)	Median (IQ Range)	
PHR (μm)	82.1 ± 3.1 (75.9–91.3)	81.7 (80.5–84.3)	81.7 ± 2.5 (75.8–86.8)	81.7 (80.2–83.6)	[a] 0.44
IRL (μm)	248.7 ± 12.4 (227.2–284.8)	246.7 (238.1–256.4)	248.3 ± 14.2 (211.6–277.4)	248.7 (237.1–258.6)	[a] 0.86
RPE (μm)	14.9 ± 1.4 (12.2–19.1)	14.8 (13.8–16.0)	14.6 ± 1.3 (11.4–17.6)	14.7 (13.6–15.6)	[a] 0.17
ONL (μm)	72.7 ± 9.1 (56.2–96.6)	70.9 (67.0–78.0)	72.9 ± 8.7 (51.9–94.6)	73.8 (66.5–79.2)	[b] 0.76
OPL (μm)	33.8 ± 4.5 (25.8–47.1)	33.8 (30.4–37.1)	33.1 ± 4.8 (25.8–45.6)	31.9 (29.3–37.0)	[b] 0.30
INL (μm)	37.5 ± 3.2 (30.4–46.3)	37.1 (35.3–39.8)	37.5 ± 3.5 (31.9–45.8)	37.3 (34.9–39.8)	[a] 0.98
IPL (μm)	39.0 ± 2.7 (32.4–45.6)	39.3 (37.6–40.4)	38.9 ± 3.0 (31.6–46.6)	38.7 (36.8–41.1)	[a] 0.88
GCL (μm)	46.5 ± 4.2 (36.3–55.7)	46.3 (43.2–49.8)	46.6 ± 4.3 (36.6–55.8)	45.9 (43.4–50.2)	[a] 0.89
RNFL (μm)	19.5 ± 1.5 (16.6–22.4)	19.6 (18.6–20.6)	19.6 ± 1.7 (16.2–24.4)	19.3 (18.2–20.6)	[a] 0.88
GCC (μm)	105.0 ± 7.5 (85.7–121.8)	105.2 (100.2–110.6)	105.1 ± 8.2 (87.0–124.3)	104.0 (99.1–112.6)	[a] 0.96
TOTAL RETINA (μm)	330.9 ± 13.8 (303.3–369.3)	329.7 (318.9–341.1)	330.0 ± 14.7 (289.0–362.1)	330.6 (319.7–338.7)	[a] 0.74

[a] Student t-test unpaired; [b] Mann Whitney U test. SD: Standard Deviation; IQ: Interquartile; PHR: Photoreceptors; IRL: Inner Retinal Layer; RPE: Retinal Pigment Epithelium; ONL: Outer Nuclear Layer; OPL: Outer Plexiform Layer; INL: Inner Nuclear Layer; IPL: Inner Plexiform Layer; GCL: Ganglion Cell Layer; RNFL: Retinal Nerve Fiber Layer; GCC: Ganglion Cell Complex.

Table 4. Comparison of total volume (mm³) between celiac patients and healthy subjects of the analyzed OCT scan.

	Celiac Patients 19 Males–47 Females		Healthy Controls 19 Males–47 Females		p-Value
	Mean ± SD (Range)	Median (IQ Range)	Mean ± SD (Range)	Median (IQ Range)	
PHR (mm³)	0.58 ± 0.02 (0.54–0.64)	0.58 (0.57–0.59)	0.58 ± 0.02 (0.53–0.61)	0.58 (0.57–0.59)	[a] 0.56
IRL (mm³)	1.77 ± 0.09 (1.61–2.02)	1.77 (1.70–1.83)	1.77 ± 0.10 (1.52–1.97)	1.77 (1.69–1.82)	[a] 0.97
RPE (mm³)	0.10 ± 0.01 (0.09–0.13)	0.10 (0.10–0.11)	0.10 ± 0.01 (0.08–0.12)	0.10 (0.10–0.11)	[a] 0.85
ONL (mm³)	0.51 ± 0.06 (0.39–0.67)	0.50 (0.47–0.55)	0.51 ± 0.06 (0.37–0.66)	0.52 (0.47–0.55)	[a] 0.74
OPL (mm³)	0.24 ± 0.03 (0.18–0.33)	0.24 (0.21–0.26)	0.23 ± 0.03 (0.18–0.32)	0.22 (0.21–0.26)	[a] 0.46
INL (mm³)	0.27 ± 0.02 (0.22–0.33)	0.27 (0.25–0.28)	0.27 ± 0.02 (0.23–0.33)	0.27 (0.25–0.28)	[a] 0.87
IPL (mm³)	0.28 ± 0.02 (0.23–0.33)	0.28 (0.27–0.29)	0.28 ± 0.02 (0.23–0.33)	0.28 (0.26–0.29)	[a] 0.60
GCL (mm³)	0.34 ± 0.03 (0.26–0.40)	0.34 (0.32–0.36)	0.34 ± 0.03 (0.27–0.40)	0.33 (0.32–0.36)	[a] 0.97
RNFL (mm³)	0.14 ± 0.01 (0.12–0.17)	0.14 (0.14–0.15)	0.14 ± 0.01 (0.12–0.18)	0.14 (0.13–0.15)	[a] 0.95
GCC (mm³)	0.76 ± 0.06 (0.62–0.90)	0.75 (0.71–0.80)	0.76 ± 0.06 (0.67–0.88)	0.75 (0.71–0.81)	[a] 0.98
TOTAL RETINA (mm³)	2.35 ± 0.10 (2.14–2.62)	2.34 (2.27–2.42)	2.34 ± 0.11 (2.07–2.57)	2.35 (2.27–2.40)	[b] 0.81

[a] Mann Whitney U test; [b] Student t-test unpaired. SD: Standard Deviation; IQ: Interquartile; PHR: Photoreceptors; IRL: Inner Retinal Layer; RPE: Retinal Pigment Epithelium; ONL: Outer Nuclear Layer; OPL: Outer Plexiform Layer; INL: Inner Nuclear Layer; IPL: Inner Plexiform Layer; GCL: Ganglion Cell Layer; RNFL: Retinal Nerve Fiber Layer; GCC: Ganglion Cell Complex.

Table 5. Comparison of peripapillary RNFL thicknesses (μm) between celiac patients and healthy subjects.

	Celiac Patients 19 Males–47 Females		Healthy Controls 19 Males–47 Females		p-Value
	Mean ± SD (Range)	Median (IQ Range)	Mean ± SD (Range)	Median (IQ Range)	
G (μm)	100.3 ± 11.5 (62.0–127.0)	102.0 (93.0–110.0)	99.5 ± 10.1 (72.0–127.0)	99.0 (94.0–104.3)	[a] 0.69
T (μm)	76.2 ± 13.1 (48.0–117.0)	75.5 (67.0–82.0)	79.4 ± 13.8 (53.0–128.0)	78.0 (69.8–90.0)	[b] 0.13
TS (μm)	133.6 ± 24.3 (42.0–190.0)	137.5 (120.0–145.5)	131.9 ± 17.8 (96.0–170.0)	133.0 (117.0–144.3)	[a] 0.64
NS (μm)	112.6 ± 23.0 (23.0–168.0)	113.0 (102.8–126.5)	105.7 ± 24.3 (39.0–171.0)	106.0 (93.8–119.0)	[a] 0.09
N (μm)	76.1 ± 14.3 (43.0–115.0)	78.0 (65.8–86.0)	74.0 ± 15.3 (40.0–123.0)	70.5 (63.8–83.3)	[b] 0.23
NI (μm)	107.4 ± 26.8 (48.0–187.0)	106.5 (88.3–124.5)	111.0 ± 28.2 (53.0–198.0)	107.5 (88.8–125.8)	[a] 0.46
TI (μm)	144.0 ± 20.9 (84.0–185.0)	142.5 (134.0–159.5)	140.9 ± 20.9 (88.0–186.0)	140.0 (129.0–157.0)	[a] 0.39

[a] Student t-test unpaired; [b] Mann Whitney U test. SD: Standard Deviation; IQ: Interquartile; G: Global average; T: Temporal; TS: Temporal-Superior; NS: Nasal-Superior; N: Nasal; NI: Nasal-Inferior; TI: Temporal-Inferior.

4. Discussion

Celiac disease is a systemic autoimmune disease that primarily affects the small intestine, although it could also present extraintestinal symptoms [22]. The eye is undoubtedly one of the disease's target organs, with dry eye, cataracts, central retinal vein occlusion, neuro-ophthalmic symptoms, night blindness, uveitis, and thyroid-associated orbitopathy all possible [23].

Considering all these possible ocular complications, an in vivo OCT analysis of the retinal layers and peripapillary RNFL trying to find possible diagnostic signs of ocular involvement in celiac disease might be helpful and of interest.

To the best of our knowledge, the present study is the first one comparing all the retinal layers and the largest one comparing peripapillary RNFL of celiac patients to a healthy control group, to highlight potential differences between the two study groups that could be explained by the underlying pathogenetic mechanisms of celiac disease.

In the present study, celiac patients showed slight diffuse thickening of almost all the retinal layers and peripapillary RNFL, with no statistically significant differences in any of the analyzed parameters.

Concerning the peripapillary RNFL, few previously published papers have addressed this issue without reaching any agreement in the results [11–14]. Our results confirmed, in adults, the findings obtained by Dereci et al. [14], who, when evaluating both peripapillary RNFL and GCC in 86 eyes of 43 children, found no significant statistical differences between celiac children and healthy controls.

On the other hand, Karatepe Hashas et al. [11] evaluated peripapillary RNFL of 31 celiac children and 34 healthy controls using SD-OCT imaging of both eyes, observing a significant overall thinning of the RNFL in celiac patients. The authors hypothesized that this finding might be attributable to autoantibodies with an affinity to retinal nerve tissue, and they also suggested further pathophysiological studies in order to verify their hypothesis.

The same hypothesis was supported by Hazar et al. [12] who, appraising peripapillary RNFL of 58 eyes of 31 celiac adults and 50 eyes of 25 healthy individuals using SD-OCT, showed a significant thinning of superior RNFL, but a significant thickening of nasal RNFL in celiac patients. Furthermore, the authors found a significant positive correlation between tissue transglutaminase autoantibody levels and the thinning of the superior RNFL, supposing an autoantibody affinity to retinal nerve tissue, as Karatepe Hashas et al. [11] found. However, no explanation on the nasal RNFL thickening was given [12].

On the other hand, Dönmez Gün et al. [13] analyzed 72 eyes of 36 celiac adults and 70 eyes of 35 age- and sex-matched healthy controls with a SD-OCT, showing an overall thinning of peripapillary RNFL in celiac patients, but without statistically significant differences between the two study groups.

Several explanations could be adduced to elucidate some differences between the previous studies [11–14] and the present one.

First, the current study utilized the largest sample size, which was determined using a power calculation assessment [21]. As a result, previous papers [11–14] may have yielded different results that contradicted one another due to small and insignificant sample sizes.

Furthermore, the present study examined just one eye per participant, whereas all prior studies [11–14] examined both eyes in some individuals and only one eye in others. According to McAlinden et al. [24,25], this might lead to statistical bias, affecting the results.

However, in the present study, no significant modification in the thicknesses of all retinal layers, especially for GCC layers, was found, confirming the findings by Dereci et al. [14]. This could make neural tissue involvement a more complicated issue [26].

The GCC is the sum of the three innermost layers: the RNFL, the ganglion cell layer (GCL), and the inner plexiform layer (IPL) [26]. The thickness of the GCC layers could be measured using SD-OCT to assess early signs of systemic and autoimmune disorders [27,28]. The thickness of the GCC layers was demonstrated to be reduced in some pathological conditions, such as systemic lupus erythematosus, Behçet's disease, obesity, and multiple sclerosis due to the impact of autoinflammatory disorders and metabolic stress [29,30].

According to the assumptions by Karatepe Hashas et al. [11] and Hazar et al. [12], the autoantibodies would cause a decrease in RNFL, GCL, and IPL, but these retinal layers seem to not be reached by these antibodies [29], even if further pathophysiological studies are needed to better understand this issue. Nevertheless, they can be affected by inflammatory processes, as it happens in the case of systemic lupus erythematosus, Behçet's disease, and multiple sclerosis. Several studies reported decreased thicknesses of the GCC layers, demonstrating that the inflammatory effects of these diseases directly influence neural tissue [29,30].

The present study's results indicate that celiac disease's inflammatory and autoimmune processes could not involve the retinal layers directly. However, this finding may also be explained by the gluten-free diet adherence of all analyzed celiac patients, possibly determining a remission of any retinal changes or a decrease in the inflammatory effects of the disease [31].

The fact that the patients were on a gluten-free diet could represent a limitation of the present study. Further studies in naïve celiac patients, comparing the effects of a gluten-free diet versus a regular diet, would be needed to understand better the retinal baseline status of such subjects and its possible changes over time.

5. Conclusions

In conclusion, retinal layer thicknesses, volumes, and peripapillary RNFL were similar in the celiac patients and the healthy individuals. The reason for these results could be due to either the non-involvement of the retinal layers in celiac disease or the gluten-free diet effect. However, the results of this study cannot omit a routine ophthalmological examination for these patients due to the association between celiac disease and other ocular disorders [4–7].

Author Contributions: M.D.B., L.V., L.E. and F.D.R. contributed to the acquisition, analysis, and interpretation of data, and also the writing of the original draft. N.R. and C.C. conceived the work and reviewed the manuscript. All authors have read and agreed to the published version of the manuscript.

Funding: The research was funded by the FARB grant from the University of Salerno.

Institutional Review Board Statement: This study was performed in line with the principles of the Declaration of Helsinki. Institutional Review Board approval was also obtained from the ComEtico Campania Sud (CECS), prot. n°16544.

Informed Consent Statement: Informed consent was obtained from all subjects involved in the study.

Data Availability Statement: The data presented in this study are available on request from the corresponding author.

Conflicts of Interest: The authors declare no conflict of interest.

References

1. Bai, J.C.; Ciacci, C. World gastroenterology organisation global guidelines: Celiac disease February 2017. *J. Clin. Gastroenterol.* **2017**, *51*, 755–768. [CrossRef] [PubMed]
2. Lindfors, K.; Ciacci, C.; Kurppa, K.; Lundin, K.E.A.; Makharia, G.K.; Mearin, M.L.; Murray, J.A.; Verdu, E.F.; Kaukinen, K. Coeliac disease. *Nat. Rev. Dis. Primers* **2019**, *5*, 3. [CrossRef] [PubMed]
3. Laurikka, P.; Nurminen, S.; Kivelä, L.; Kurppa, K. Extraintestinal manifestations of celiac disease: Early detection for better long-term outcomes. *Nutrients* **2018**, *10*, 1015. [CrossRef] [PubMed]
4. Bolukbasi, S.; Erden, B.; Cakir, A.; Bayat, A.H.; Elcioglu, M.N.; Ocak, S.Y.; Gokden, Y.; Adas, M.; Asik, Z.N. Pachychoroid pigment epitheliopathy and choroidal thickness changes in coeliac disease. *J. Ophthalmol.* **2019**, *2019*, 6924191. [CrossRef]
5. Uzel, M.M.; Citirik, M.; Kekilli, M.; Cicek, P. Local ocular surface parameters in patients with systemic celiac disease. *Eye* **2017**, *31*, 1093–1098. [CrossRef] [PubMed]
6. Al Hemidan, A.I.; Tabbara, K.F.; Althomali, T. Vogt-Koyanagi-Harada associated with diabetes mellitus and celiac disease in a 3-year-old girl. *Eur. J. Ophthalmol.* **2006**, *16*, 173–177. [CrossRef]
7. Mollazadegan, K.; Kugelberg, M.; Lindblad, B.E.; Ludvigsson, J.F. Increased risk of cataract among 28,000 patients with celiac disease. *Am. J. Epidemiol.* **2011**, *174*, 195–202. [CrossRef]
8. Doğan, G.; Şen, S.; Çavdar, E.; Mayalı, H.; Özyurt, B.C.; Kurt, E.; Kasırga, E. Should we worry about the eyes of celiac patients? *Eur. J. Ophthalmol.* **2020**, *30*, 886–890. [CrossRef]
9. De Bernardo, M.; Vitiello, L.; Battipaglia, M.; Mascolo, F.; Iovino, C.; Capasso, L.; Ciacci, C.; Rosa, N. Choroidal structural evaluation in celiac disease. *Sci. Rep.* **2021**, *11*, 16398. [CrossRef] [PubMed]
10. De Bernardo, M.; Vitiello, L.; Gagliardi, M.; Capasso, L.; Rosa, N.; Ciacci, C. Ocular anterior segment and corneal parameters evaluation in celiac disease. *Sci. Rep.* **2022**, *12*, 2203. [CrossRef]
11. Karatepe Hashas, A.S.; Altunel, O.; Sevınc, E.; Duru, N.; Alabay, B.; Torun, Y.A. The eyes of children with celiac disease. *J. Am. Assoc. Pediatr. Ophthalmol. Strabismus* **2017**, *21*, 48–51. [CrossRef] [PubMed]
12. Hazar, L.; Oyur, G.; Atay, K. Evaluation of ocular parameters in adult patients with celiac disease. *Curr. Eye Res.* **2021**, *46*, 122–126. [CrossRef] [PubMed]
13. Dönmez Gün, R.; Kaplan, A.T.; Zorlutuna Kaymak, N.; Köroğlu, E.; Karadağ, E.; Şimşek, Ş. The impact of celiac disease and duration of gluten free diet on anterior and posterior ocular structures: Ocular imaging based study. *Photodiagnosis Photodyn. Ther.* **2021**, *34*, 102214. [CrossRef] [PubMed]
14. Dereci, S.; Asik, A.; Direkci, I.; Karadag, A.S.; Hizli, S. Evaluation of eye involvement in paediatric celiac disease patients. *Int. J. Clin. Pract.* **2021**, *75*, e14679. [CrossRef]
15. De Bernardo, M.; Capasso, L.; Caliendo, L.; Vosa, Y.; Rosa, N. Intraocular pressure evaluation after myopic refractive surgery: A comparison of methods in 121 eyes. *Semin. Ophthalmol.* **2016**, *31*, 233–242. [CrossRef] [PubMed]
16. Rosa, N.; Cione, F.; Pepe, A.; Musto, S.; De Bernardo, M. An Advanced Lens Measurement Approach (ALMA) in post refractive surgery IOL power calculation with unknown preoperative parameters. *PLoS ONE* **2020**, *15*, e0237990. [CrossRef] [PubMed]
17. De Bernardo, M.; Capasso, L.; Caliendo, L.; Paolercio, F.; Rosa, N. IOL power calculation after corneal refractive surgery. *Biomed. Res. Int.* **2014**, *2014*, 658350. [CrossRef] [PubMed]
18. De Bernardo, M.; Salerno, G.; Cornetta, P.; Rosa, N. Axial length shortening after cataract surgery: New approach to solve the question. *Transl. Vis. Sci. Technol.* **2018**, *7*, 34. [CrossRef] [PubMed]
19. Murdoch, I.E.; Morris, S.S.; Cousens, S.N. People and eyes: Statistical approaches in ophthalmology. *Br. J. Ophthalmol.* **1998**, *82*, 971–973. [CrossRef] [PubMed]
20. Kim, B.J.; Irwin, D.J.; Song, D.; Daniel, E.; Leveque, J.D.; Raquib, A.R.; Pan, W.; Ying, G.-S.; Aleman, T.S.; Dunaief, J.L.; et al. Optical coherence tomography identifies outer retina thinning in frontotemporal degeneration. *Neurology* **2017**, *89*, 1604–1611. [CrossRef]
21. Faul, F.; Erdfelder, E.; Lang, A.G.; Buchner, A. G*Power 3: A flexible statistical power analysis program for the social, behavioral, and biomedical sciences. *Behav. Res. Methods* **2007**, *39*, 175–191. [CrossRef] [PubMed]
22. Ludvigsson, J.F.; Bai, J.C.; Biagi, F.; Card, T.R.; Ciacci, C.; Ciclitira, P.J.; Green, P.H.R.; Hadjivassiliou, M.; Holdoway, A.; van Heel, D.A.; et al. BSG Coeliac Disease Guidelines Development Group; British Society of Gastroenterology. Diagnosis and management of adult coeliac disease: Guidelines from the British Society of Gastroenterology. *Gut* **2014**, *63*, 1210–1228. [CrossRef] [PubMed]

23. Fousekis, F.S.; Katsanos, A.; Katsanos, K.H.; Christodoulou, D.K. Ocular manifestations in celiac disease: An overview. *Int. Ophthalmol.* **2020**, *40*, 1049–1054. [CrossRef]
24. McAlinden, C.; Khadka, J.; Pesudovs, K. Statistical methods for conducting agreement (comparison of clinical tests) and precision (repeatability or reproducibility) studies in optometry and ophthalmology. *Ophthalmic Physiol. Opt.* **2011**, *31*, 330–338. [CrossRef]
25. McAlinden, C.; Khadka, J.; Pesudovs, K. Precision (repeatability and reproducibility) studies and sample-size calculation. *J. Cataract. Refract. Surg.* **2015**, *41*, 2598–2604. [CrossRef]
26. Hormel, T.T.; Jia, Y.; Jian, Y.; Hwang, T.S.; Bailey, S.T.; Pennesi, M.E.; Wilson, D.J.; Morrison, J.C.; Huang, D. Plexus-specific retinal vascular anatomy and pathologies as seen by projection-resolved optical coherence tomographic angiography. *Prog. Retin. Eye Res.* **2021**, *80*, 100878. [CrossRef]
27. Duru, N.; Altinkaynak, H.; Erten, Ş.; Can, M.E.; Duru, Z.; Uğurlu, F.G.; Çağıl, N. Thinning of choroidal thickness in patients with rheumatoid arthritis unrelated to disease activity. *Ocul. Immunol. Inflamm.* **2016**, *24*, 246–253. [CrossRef]
28. Ishikawa, S.; Taguchi, M.; Muraoka, T.; Sakurai, Y.; Kanda, T.; Takeuchi, M. Changes in subfoveal choroidal thickness associated with uveitis activity in patients with Behçet's disease. *Br. J. Ophthalmol.* **2014**, *98*, 1508–1513. [CrossRef]
29. Saidha, S.; Syc, S.B.; Durbin, M.K.; Eckstein, C.; Oakley, J.D.; Meyer, S.A.; Conger, A.; Frohman, T.C.; Newsome, S.; Ratchford, J.N.; et al. Visual dysfunction in multiple sclerosis correlates better with optical coherence tomography derived estimates of macular ganglion cell layer thickness than peripapillary retinal nerve fiber layer thickness. *Mult. Scler.* **2011**, *17*, 1449–1463. [CrossRef]
30. Karti, O.; Nalbantoglu, O.; Abali, S.; Tunc, S.; Ozkan, B. The assessment of peripapillary retinal nerve fiber layer and macular ganglion cell layer changes in obese children: A crosssectional study using optical coherence tomography. *Int. Ophthalmol.* **2017**, *37*, 1031–1038. [CrossRef]
31. Rubio-Tapia, A.; Hill, I.D.; Kelly, C.P.; Calderwood, A.H.; Murray, J.A.; American College of Gastroenterology. ACG clinical guidelines: Diagnosis and management of celiac disease. *Am. J. Gastroenterol.* **2013**, *108*, 656–676. [CrossRef] [PubMed]

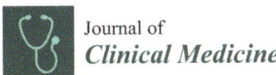

Article

Anatomical and Functional Effects of Oral Administration of Curcuma Longa and Boswellia Serrata Combination in Patients with Treatment-Naïve Diabetic Macular Edema

Olimpia Guarino [1,†], Claudio Iovino [1,*,†], Valentina Di Iorio [1], Andrea Rosolia [1], Irene Schiavetti [2], Michele Lanza [1] and Francesca Simonelli [1]

1 Eye Clinic, Multidisciplinary Department of Medical, Surgical and Dental Sciences, University of Campania Luigi Vanvitelli, 80131 Naples, Italy; olimpia.guarino@hotmail.it (O.G.); valentina.diiorio@unicampania.it (V.D.I.); dr.rosolia@gmail.com (A.R.); mic.lanza@gmail.com (M.L.); francesca.simonelli@unicampania.it (F.S.)
2 Department of Health Sciences, University of Genoa, 16132 Genoa, Italy; irene.schiavetti@unige.it
* Correspondence: claudio.iovino1@unicampania.it
† These authors contributed equally to this work.

Abstract: Anti-vascular endothelial growth factor nowdays represents the standard of care for diabetic macular edema (DME). Nevertheless, the burden of injections worldwide has created tremendous stress on the healthcare system during the COVID-19 pandemic. The aim of this study was to investigate the effects of the oral administration of Curcuma longa and Boswellia serrata (Retimix®) in patients with non-proliferative diabetic retinopathy (DR) and treatment-naïve DME < 400 µm, managed during the COVID-19 pandemic. In this retrospective study, patients were enrolled and divided into two groups, one undergoing observation (Group A, n 12) and one receiving one sachet a day of Retimix® (Group B, n 49). Best-corrected visual acuity (BCVA) and central macular thickness (CMT) measured by spectral-domain optical coherence tomography were performed at baseline, then at one and six months. A mixed-design ANOVA was calculated to determine whether the change in CMT and BCVA over time differed according to the consumption of Retimix®. The interaction between time and treatment was significant, with F (1.032, 102.168) = 14.416; η^2 = 0.127; $p < 0.001$, indicating that the change in terms of CMT and BCVA over time among groups was significantly different. In conclusion, our results show the efficacy of Curcuma longa and Boswellia serrata in patients with non-proliferative DR and treatment-naïve DME in maintaining baseline CMT and BCVA values over time.

Keywords: Boswellia serrata; curcumin; diabetic macular edema

1. Introduction

Diabetic retinopathy (DR) is one of the main causes of working-age visual loss in industrialized countries. It is a long-term manifestation of diabetic microangiopathy which most commonly affects the eyes, the peripheral nerves, and the kidneys [1]. DR is caused by damage to the retinal blood vessels that affects the macular region and the peripheral retina, resulting in an overall reduction of visual function [1].

Diabetic macular edema (DME) is the result of intraretinal fluid accumulation in extracellular location, due to the breakdown of the blood-retinal barrier [2]. This process is caused by the release of pro-inflammatory substances. Hyperglycemia stimulates a hyper-activation of microglia with the consequent development of the inflammatory process mediated by interleukin (IL)-1β, tumor necrosis factor (TNF)-α, IL-6, and vascular endothelial growth factor (VEGF) [3]. In concomitance, the alteration of ion exchanges between photoreceptors and Müller cells creates a fluid overflow with the formation of intracellular edema. The production of VEGF molecules contributes to increased vascular permeability and thus vascular homeostasis loss [4].

DME formation can occur in both the proliferative and non-proliferative forms of DR and its onset is typically associated with some characteristic symptoms, including visual blurring and distorted vision. Fluorescein angiography (FA), through the detection of macular capillary hyperpermeability, and optical coherence tomography (OCT), through the detection of intra and subretinal fluid, represent the specific diagnostic investigations currently used to detect DME [5,6].

According to the current literature, when DME is considered subclinical for its size and localization and is associated with a good visual acuity, the patient can be monitored over time with no treatment administered [7,8].

There are some natural substances, not considered to be medications, that have been shown to help in the treatment of systemic and ocular pathological conditions [9–11]. Among these, the root of Curcuma longa, rich in polyphenols, is a potent anti-inflammatory agent and prevents the formation of reactive oxygen species. The latter can lead to pathological processes, like cell apoptosis, angiogenesis, and inflammation ending in retinal pathologies [12].

Boswellic acids derived from the gum of the Boswellia serrata (a plant native to India) also have anti-inflammatory and anti-arthritic activities [13,14]. Recent studies have shown that the association of active ingredients derived from Curcuma longa and Boswellia serrata acts synergistically to counteract the pathways of inflammation at multiple levels [15,16].

Retimix®, a combination of the two described substances, would allow for the exploitation of the combined and synergistic activity of its components in the control of the inflammatory processes occurring in retinal disorders, including DR.

On this background, the aim of this study was to investigate the anatomical and functional effects of the oral administration of Curcuma longa and Boswellia serrata in patients with non-proliferative DR and treatment-naïve DME, managed during the COVID-19 pandemic.

2. Methods

In this study, patients with treatment-naïve DME managed during the COVID-19 pandemic were retrospectively evaluated at the Retina Unit of the University of Campania "Luigi Vanvitelli". Institutional review board approval was obtained for a retrospective consecutive chart review by the Vanvitelli University Ethics Committee. The study adhered to the guidelines of the Health Insurance Portability and Accountability Act and was performed in accordance with the tenets of the Declaration of Helsinki.

Inclusion criteria were: patients with type 2 diabetes treated indifferently with antidiabetic therapy based on metformin or insulin, having non-proliferative DR with DME and central macular thickness (CMT) < 400 μm. Diagnosis of DR and DME was based on patients' history and multimodal imaging evaluation including fundus color picture, FA and spectral-domain (SD)-OCT. All patients were treatment-naïve and were enrolled during the COVID-19 pandemic under public health restrictions, with limitations in terms of operating rooms available and daily scheduled visits.

The exclusion criteria were: the presence of any other retinal disease or ocular disorder that could be associated with the development of macular edema (e.g., recent history of cataract and/or vitreoretinal surgery in the previous 6 months), hyperopia or myopia > 6 diopters, and any other concomitant nutritional supplements therapy. Additionally, patients with media opacities that could influence image quality were also excluded from the study.

Subjects who met all inclusion criteria were enrolled in the study and divided in two groups, one undergoing observation (Group A) and one receiving Retimix® (Group B). A detailed systemic and ocular history was obtained and patients underwent a complete ocular examination at each visit, including Best-Corrected Visual Acuity (BCVA) testing using 4-m ETDRS charts, slit-lamp biomicroscopy, intraocular pressure evaluation with Goldmann applanation tonometry, and CMT measurement by SD-OCT (Cirrus 4000, Carl Zeiss Meditec, Dublin, CA, USA). The overall treatment duration was 6 months and data were collected at baseline (T_0), 1 month (T_1), and 6 months (T_2). All OCT scans were acquired with follow-up function.

Group B patients received one sachet a day of Retimix® formulation which contains Casperiva®, EyePharma, corresponding to demethoxycurcumin and bisdemethoxycurcumin plus Boswellic acid in phosphatidylcholine phytosome for a total of 0.5 g phospholipidic-complex; one single foil pouch of powder per day.

All patients were also followed by a diabetologist, to ascertain a good metabolic control.

Anatomical and functional changes, in terms of CMT reduction and BCVA improvement, were evaluated over time and compared between the two groups. The percentage of patients having systemic hypertension and dyslipidemia were also recorded.

Statistical Methods

Continuous variables are summarized as mean with standard, and categorical data are expressed with frequency and percentage.

A mixed-design ANOVA was calculated to determine whether the change of CMT and BCVA over time (from baseline to 1 month and 6 months) differed according to the consumption of Retimix® formulation. In particular, the model included time as a within-subject factor, and sex, CMT, and treatment group as a between-subject factor. Age and BCVA at baseline were included in the analysis as covariates.

For data which violated the normal distribution, p-values were adjusted using the Greenhouse–Geisser correction, and the adjusted p-values were reported.

Alpha for statistical test was set at 0.05.

3. Results

Sixty-one (61) patients, 31 females (50.8%) and 30 males (49.2%) with a mean age of 64.2 (±14.13) years old, were enrolled and divided in two groups: observation (Group A, n = 12) and treatment (Group B, n = 49).

All baseline demographic and clinical ocular and systemic characteristics of the total cohort are summarized in Table 1.

Table 1. Baseline demographic and clinical ocular and systemic characteristics of study patients.

		Total N = 61	Group A N = 12	Group B N = 49	p
Age (years)		64.2 ± 14.13	65.8 ± 17.76	63.8 ± 13.23	0.44
Sex	Female	31(50.8)	7 (58.3)	24 (49.0)	0.56
	Male	30 (49.2)	5 (41.7)	25 (51.0)	
CMT (μm) at baseline		276.3 ± 72.80	291.6 ± 47.63	272.6 (77.67)	0.09
BCVA (ETDRS Letters)		52.9 ± 14.60	51.7 ± 18.78	53.2 (13.61)	0.82
Systemic hypertension		32 (52.5)	7 (58.3)	25 (51.0)	0.65
Dyslipidemia		8 (13.1)	2 (16.7)	6 (12.2)	0.68
Pseudophakia		18 (29.5)	3 (25.0)	15 (30.6)	0.70

BCVA = best-corrected visual acuity; CMT = central macular thickness.

There were no statistically significant differences in the two groups regarding demographics, ocular (BCVA, CMT, pseudophakia), and systemic parameters (systemic hypertension and dyslipidemia) at baseline evaluation. No patients received either pars plana vitrectomy or retinal laser treatments before the inclusion or during the study.

The mixed-model ANOVA showed that time alone had a non-significant main effect: the CMT at the end of the follow-ups was not significantly different in the two groups from that at the beginning of the study in the total cohort, $F (1.032, 102.168) = 0.107$; $\eta^2 = 0.001$ ($p = 0.75$).

Likewise, the main effect of group on the size of CMT (regardless of the time) was not significant, $F (1, 99) = 3.862$; $\eta^2 = 0.038$; $p = 0.052$.

Conversely, the interaction between time and treatment was significant, with F (1.032,102.168) = 14.416; η^2 = 0.127 ($p < 0.001$), indicating that the change in CMT among groups was significantly different (Table 2).

Table 2. Central macular thickness changes over time.

	Baseline	One Month	Six Months	Mixed-Model ANOVA
Group A	289.91 (14.79)	289.92 (14.78)	394.22 (14.66)	F (1.032,102.168) = 14.416; η^2 = 0.127; $p < 0.001$
Group B	263.50 (7.61)	263.89 (7.60)	260.30 (7.54)	

Results are expressed as estimated marginal mean with standard error. Covariates appearing in the model are evaluated at the following values: Age, years = 63.697, Visus at baseline = 53.377.

Specifically, there was no overall natural change in CMT over time, but there was a significant reduction of CMT in patients of Group B at six months (Figure 1).

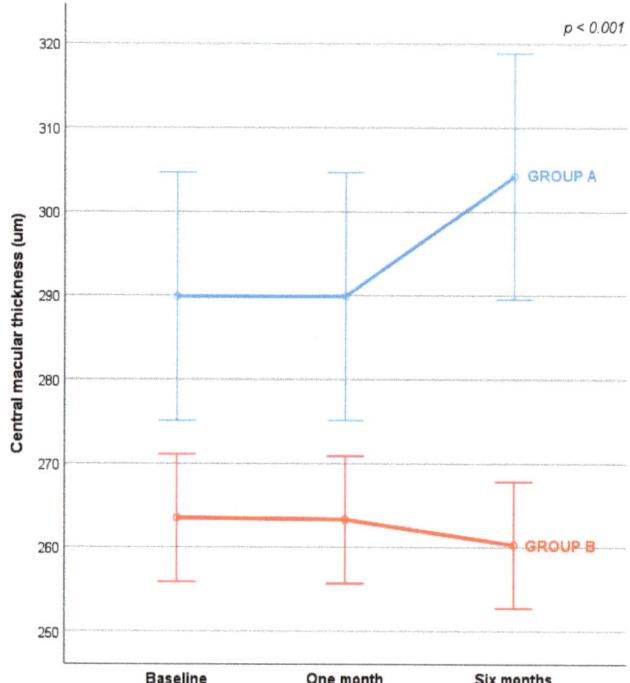

Figure 1. Central macular thickness changes over time. Covariates appearing in the model are evaluated at the following values: Age, years = 63.697, T_0 Visus = 53.377. Error bars: +/−1 SE.

After the first month of treatment both groups remained mostly stable. After six months there was a significant difference between the groups: Group B in particular remained unchanged compared to Group A, which showed a worsening in CMT dimension.

The interaction between time and treatment on BCVA was also significant, F (1.084, 108.386) = 12.514; η^2 = 0.111; $p < 0.001$, indicating that the change in BCVA among groups was significantly different (Table 3).

Table 3. Best-corrected visual acuity changes over time.

	Baseline	One Month	Six Months	Mixed-Model ANOVA
Group A	53.14 (3.60)	53.14 (3.59)	50.50 (3.69)	$F_{(1.084, 108.386)} = 12.514$; $\eta^2 = 0.111$; $p < 0.001$
Group B	53.75 (1.85)	53.70 (1.85)	54.44 (1.90)	

Results are expressed as estimated marginal mean with standard error. Covariates appearing in the model are evaluated at the following values: Age, years = 63.697.

4. Discussion

DME is the most prevalent vision-threatening complication of DR, particularly among adults with type 2 diabetes [17]. Although anti-VEFG nowadays represents the standard of care, the burden of injections worldwide has posed a tremendous stress to the healthcare system.

During the COVID-19 pandemic, the postponement of appointments and treatments in non-monocular patients with DME was proposed [18].

Recently, data from the DRCR Protocol V randomized clinical trial suggest that it is safe to observe patients with centre-involved DME and good vision (20/25 or better). Overall, a total of 702 patients were managed with either laser, aflibercept, or observation, and at 2 years the mean BCVA was 20/20 in all three cohorts [7].

In a subanalysis of the RESTORE study, patients were stratified by baseline central retinal thickness (CRT < 300 µm, 300–400 µm, and >400 µm). Among patients treated with ranibizumab greater gains in BCVA were achieved in patients with a higher baseline CRT [19].

Similarly, results from the Protocol I study, suggest that ranibizumab treated patients with DME with higher baseline central subfield thickness (CST; ≥400 µm) achieved greater visual gains.

On this background, the aim of our study was to investigate the anatomical and functional effects of the oral administration of Curcuma longa and Boswellia serrata in patients with treatment-naïve DME, managed during COVID-19 pandemic.

Public restrictions limited the number of intravitreal injections performed and the number of visits for all patients including diabetic patients. Following the published guidelines for intravitreal injections during the pandemic [18], we postponed non-urgent cases and decided to treat with anti-VEGF injections only patients having DME > 400 µm. Our results showed that patients receiving one sachet of oral Retimix® did not show a significant change in CMT at six months when compared to patients undergoing observation.

The specific characteristics of the Retimix® active ingredients, combined with the actions described above, make them an ideal agent as a preventive treatment in many pathologies due to inflammatory and vascular factors, as for DR.

The Casperiva (Retimix®) formula consists of curcuminoids, the main one being curcumin, together with demethoxycurcumin and bisdemethoxycurcumin. Among the active ingredients extracted for the formulation there are also several boswellic acids, belonging to the triterpenoid family; AKBA (3-Acetyl-11-keto-beta-Boswellic Acid) is the most documented and active [15].

Recent studies have shown that curcumin is implicated in the functions of natural responses to inflammation, both with a direct action on metabolic pathways, and on the enzymes expression level, transcription factors, and cytokines, through the suppression of the activation of the nuclear inflammatory transcription factor NF-kB, which regulates the expression of the genes of pro-inflammatory cytokines (IL-1, IL-6, TNFα), and secondly "downregulates" the expression of COX-2 (cyclooxygenase-2) [20].

One of the action mechanisms of the substance is its ability to induce peroxisome proliferator-activetedreceptor gamma (PPAR-γ) activation. PPARs play an important role in lipid degeneration, immune regulation, the control of reactive oxygen species (ROS) and VEGF, matrix metalloproteinases-9 (MMP-9), and docosahexaenoic acid (DHA). In addition, PPAR gamma is expressed in RPE cells.

Boswellic acids such as 11-keto-β-boswellic acid (KBA) and its acetylated counterpart (AKBA) have been proposed as selective inhibitors of 5-lipoxygenase (5-LO) because they regulate the inflammatory response function through the inhibition of leukotrienes. Boswellic acids have an action on 5-LO, inhibiting leukotrienes, which increase vascular permeability, as well as mast cells and histamine release and neutrophil recall [21]. In particular, AKBA has been shown to have a proven direct inhibitory action on VEGF.

The action of curcuminoids on VEGF, therefore, is indirect, because it passes through PPAR-γ, whereas AKBA has a direct action on VEGF expression. This allows a dual action both on VEGF and neo angiogenesis, and on the inflammation control to which the tissue is subjected, with a control of the inflammatory process at multiple levels [22].

The limits of the bioavailability of natural extracts, and therefore of their therapeutic efficacy, have been overcome thanks to the patented Phytosome® technology. This technology encloses the active ingredients in a new phospholipidic complex (phosphaditilserine and phosphaditilcholine) developed by Eye Pharma SpA—Genova, Italy, in collaboration with Indena SpA—Milan, Italy that protects them from gastric degradation with a complete absorption in the intestine [23–25]. All these molecular characteristics of these active ingredients built the rationale for us to use Retimix® in the management of treatment-naïve diabetic patients with DME who could not receive intravitreal injections or laser treatment due to COVID-19 pandemic restrictions. The main limitations of our study include its retrospective nature and the relatively small number of patients included. Nevertheless, this was not an impediment for the statistical analysis.

In conclusion, our results suggest the protective role of the oral administration of Curcuma longa and Boswellia serrata in patients with non-proliferative DR and treatment-naïve DME in maintaining baseline CMT and BCVA values over time. Considering its anti-inflammatory and anti-angiogenic properties, the Retimix® formulation could be also considered as an adjuvant therapy for patients with DME receiving intravitreal injections, but this awaits further prospective validation.

Author Contributions: Conceptualization, O.G., C.I. and F.S.; methodology, O.G. and C.I.; writing—original draft preparation, O.G., M.L., C.I. and I.S., writing—review and editing, M.L., O.G, C.I., V.D.I., A.R., I.S. and F.S.; supervision, C.I. and F.S. All authors have read and agreed to the published version of the manuscript.

Funding: This research received no external funding.

Institutional Review Board Statement: The study was conducted in accordance with the Declaration of Helsinki, and approved by the Institutional Review Board of Vanvitelli University Ethics Committee.

Informed Consent Statement: Informed consent was obtained from all subjects involved in the study.

Data Availability Statement: Not applicable.

Conflicts of Interest: The authors declare no conflict of interest.

References

1. Bandello, F.; Battaglia Parodi, M.; Lanzetta, P.; Loewenstein, A.; Massin, P.; Menchini, F.; Veritti, D. Diabetic Macular Edema. *Dev. Ophthalmol.* **2017**, *58*, 102–138. [CrossRef] [PubMed]
2. Starace, V.; Battista, M.; Brambati, M.; Cavalleri, M.; Bertuzzi, F.; Amato, A.; Lattanzio, R.; Bandello, F.; Cicinelli, M.V. The Role of Inflammation and Neurodegeneration in Diabetic Macular Edema. *Ther. Adv. Ophthalmol.* **2021**, *13*, 251584142110559. [CrossRef] [PubMed]
3. Noma, H.; Yasuda, K.; Shimura, M. Involvement of Cytokines in the Pathogenesis of Diabetic Macular Edema. *Int. J. Mol. Sci.* **2021**, *22*, 3427. [CrossRef]
4. Romero-Aroca, P.; Baget-Bernaldiz, M.; Pareja-Rios, A.; Lopez-Galvez, M.; Navarro-Gil, R.; Verges, R. Diabetic Macular Edema Pathophysiology: Vasogenic versus Inflammatory. *J. Diabetes Res.* **2016**, *2016*, 2156273. [CrossRef]
5. Georgiadou, E.; Moschos, M.M.; Margetis, I.; Chalkiadakis, J.; Markomichelakis, N.N. Structural and Functional Outcomes after Treatment of Uveitic Macular Oedema: An Optical Coherence Tomography and Multifocal Electroretinogram Study. *Clin. Exp. Optom.* **2012**, *95*, 89–93. [CrossRef]

6. Elsharkawy, M.; Elrazzaz, M.; Sharafeldeen, A.; Alhalabi, M.; Khalifa, F.; Soliman, A.; Elnakib, A.; Mahmoud, A.; Ghazal, M.; El-Daydamony, E.; et al. The Role of Different Retinal Imaging Modalities in Predicting Progression of Diabetic Retinopathy: A Survey. *Sensors* **2022**, *22*, 3490. [CrossRef] [PubMed]
7. Baker, C.W.; Glassman, A.R.; Beaulieu, W.T.; Antoszyk, A.N.; Browning, D.J.; Chalam, K.V.; Grover, S.; Jampol, L.M.; Jhaveri, C.D.; Melia, M.; et al. Effect of Initial Management with Aflibercept vs Laser Photocoagulation vs. Observation on Vision Loss Among Patients with Diabetic Macular Edema Involving the Center of the Macula and Good Visual Acuity. *JAMA* **2019**, *321*, 1880. [CrossRef]
8. Busch, C.; Fraser-Bell, S.; Zur, D.; Rodríguez-Valdés, P.J.; Cebeci, Z.; Lupidi, M.; Fung, A.T.; Gabrielle, P.-H.; Giancipoli, E.; Chaikitmongkol, V.; et al. Real-World Outcomes of Observation and Treatment in Diabetic Macular Edema with Very Good Visual Acuity: The OBTAIN Study. *Acta Diabetol.* **2019**, *56*, 777–784. [CrossRef]
9. Huynh, T.-P.; Mann, S.N.; Mandal, N.A. Botanical Compounds: Effects on Major Eye Diseases. *Evid. Based Complement. Altern. Med.* **2013**, *2013*, 549174. [CrossRef]
10. Pescosolido, N.; Giannotti, R.; Plateroti, A.; Pascarella, A.; Nebbioso, M. Curcumin: Therapeutical Potential in Ophthalmology. *Planta Med.* **2013**, *80*, 249–254. [CrossRef] [PubMed]
11. Peddada, K.V.; Brown, A.; Verma, V.; Nebbioso, M. Therapeutic Potential of Curcumin in Major Retinal Pathologies. *Int. Ophthalmol.* **2019**, *39*, 725–734. [CrossRef]
12. López-Malo, D.; Villarón-Casares, C.A.; Alarcón-Jiménez, J.; Miranda, M.; Díaz-Llopis, M.; Romero, F.J.; Villar, V.M. Curcumin as a Therapeutic Option in Retinal Diseases. *Antioxidants* **2020**, *9*, 48. [CrossRef] [PubMed]
13. Ammon, H. Boswellic Acids in Chronic Inflammatory Diseases. *Planta Med.* **2006**, *72*, 1100–1116. [CrossRef] [PubMed]
14. Ammon, H.P.T. Modulation of the Immune System by Boswellia Serrata Extracts and Boswellic Acids. *Phytomedicine* **2010**, *17*, 862–867. [CrossRef]
15. Ammon, H.P.T.; Safayhi, H.; Mack, T.; Sabieraj, J. Mechanism of Antiinflammatory Actions of Curcumine and Boswellic Acids. *J. Ethnopharmacol.* **1993**, *38*, 105–112. [CrossRef]
16. Haroyan, A.; Mukuchyan, V.; Mkrtchyan, N.; Minasyan, N.; Gasparyan, S.; Sargsyan, A.; Narimanyan, M.; Hovhannisyan, A. Efficacy and Safety of Curcumin and Its Combination with Boswellic Acid in Osteoarthritis: A Comparative, Randomized, Double-Blind, Placebo-Controlled Study. *BMC Complement. Altern. Med.* **2018**, *18*, 7. [CrossRef]
17. Tan, G.S.; Cheung, N.; Simó, R.; Cheung, G.C.M.; Wong, T.Y. Diabetic Macular Oedema. *Lancet Diabetes Endocrinol.* **2017**, *5*, 143–155. [CrossRef]
18. Korobelnik, J.-F.; Loewenstein, A.; Eldem, B.; Joussen, A.M.; Koh, A.; Lambrou, G.N.; Lanzetta, P.; Li, X.; Lövestam-Adrian, M.; Navarro, R.; et al. Guidance for Anti-VEGF Intravitreal Injections during the COVID-19 Pandemic. *Graefe's Arch. Clin. Exp. Ophthalmol.* **2020**, *258*, 1149–1156. [CrossRef]
19. Mitchell, P.; Bandello, F.; Schmidt-Erfurth, U.; Lang, G.E.; Massin, P.; Schlingemann, R.O.; Sutter, F.; Simader, C.; Burian, G.; Gerstner, O.; et al. The RESTORE Study. *Ophthalmology* **2011**, *118*, 615–625. [CrossRef] [PubMed]
20. He, Y.; Yue, Y.; Zheng, X.; Zhang, K.; Chen, S.; Du, Z. Curcumin, Inflammation, and Chronic Diseases: How Are They Linked? *Molecules* **2015**, *20*, 9183–9213. [CrossRef]
21. Loeser, K.; Seemann, S.; König, S.; Lenhardt, I.; Abdel-Tawab, M.; Koeberle, A.; Werz, O.; Lupp, A. Protective Effect of Casperome®, an Orally Bioavailable Frankincense Extract, on Lipopolysaccharide- Induced Systemic Inflammation in Mice. *Front. Pharmacol.* **2018**, *9*, 387. [CrossRef] [PubMed]
22. Lulli, M.; Cammalleri, M.; Fornaciari, I.; Casini, G.; Dal Monte, M. Acetyl-11-Keto-β-Boswellic Acid Reduces Retinal Angiogenesis in a Mouse Model of Oxygen-Induced Retinopathy. *Exp. Eye Res.* **2015**, *135*, 67–80. [CrossRef]
23. Cuomo, J.; Appendino, G.; Dern, A.S.; Schneider, E.; McKinnon, T.P.; Brown, M.J.; Togni, S.; Dixon, B.M. Comparative Absorption of a Standardized Curcuminoid Mixture and Its Lecithin Formulation. *J. Nat. Prod.* **2011**, *74*, 664–669. [CrossRef]
24. Riva, A.; Morazzoni, P.; Artaria, C.; Allegrini, P.; Meins, J.; Savio, D.; Appendino, G.; Schubert-Zsilavecz, M.; Abdel-Tawab, M. A Single-Dose, Randomized, Cross-over, Two-Way, Open-Label Study for Comparing the Absorption of Boswellic Acids and Its Lecithin Formulation. *Phytomedicine* **2016**, *23*, 1375–1382. [CrossRef]
25. Hüsch, J.; Bohnet, J.; Fricker, G.; Skarke, C.; Artaria, C.; Appendino, G.; Schubert-Zsilavecz, M.; Abdel-Tawab, M. Enhanced Absorption of Boswellic Acids by a Lecithin Delivery Form (Phytosome®) of Boswellia Extract. *Fitoterapia* **2013**, *84*, 89–98. [CrossRef]

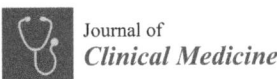

Article

Early Structural and Vascular Changes after Within-24 Hours Vitrectomy for Recent Onset Rhegmatogenous Retinal Detachment Treatment: A Pilot Study Comparing Bisected Macula and Not Bisected Macula

Rossella D'Aloisio [1,*,†], Matteo Gironi [2,†], Tommaso Verdina [2], Chiara Vivarelli [2], Riccardo Leonelli [2], Cesare Mariotti [3], Shaniko Kaleci [4], Lisa Toto [1] and Rodolfo Mastropasqua [1]

[1] Ophthalmology Clinic, Department of Medicine and Science of Ageing, University Gabriele D'Annunzio Chieti-Pescara, 66100 Chieti, Italy; l.toto@unich.it (L.T.); rodolfo.mastropasqua@gmail.com (R.M.)
[2] Ophthalmology Clinic, Azienda Ospedaliero-Universitaria di Modena, University of Modena and Reggio Emilia, 41122 Modena, Italy; matteo.gironi@hotmail.it (M.G.); tommaso.verdina@gmail.com (T.V.); chia.vivarelli@gmail.com (C.V.); leoneliriccardo@outlook.it (R.L.)
[3] Eye Clinic, AOU Ospedali Riuniti Ancona-Polytechnic University of Marche, 60121 Ancona, Italy; cesare.mariotti@ospedaliriuniti.marche.it
[4] Department of Surgical, Medical, Dental and Morphological Sciences with Interest Transplant, Oncological and Regenerative Medicine, Azienda Ospedaliero-Universitaria di Modena, University of Modena and Reggio Emilia, 41122 Modena, Italy; shaniko.kaleci@unimore.it
* Correspondence: ross.daloisio@gmail.com
† These authors contributed equally to this work and should be considered as co-first authors.

Abstract: Background: In this study we aimed at investigating macular perfusion/anatomical changes in eyes with early onset rhegmatogenous retinal detachment (RRD) after prompt surgery within 24 h, comparing a bisected macula and not bisected macula RRD. Methods: In this prospective observational study, 14 eyes of 14 patients who underwent within-24 hours vitreoretinal surgery for early onset RRD were enrolled. Patients were further divided into two subgroups: the not bisected macula group (NBM group) and the bisected macula group (BM group). At baseline and 3-month follow up, macular architecture and vessel analysis were assessed using optical coherence tomography angiography (OCTA) imaging. In detail, quantitative and qualitative analyses of the macular area were performed to quantify topographical retinal perfusion changes after surgery, calculating the foveal avascular zone (FAZ), vessel density (VD) and vessel length density (VLD) at the superficial capillary plexus (SCP) and deep capillary plexus (DCP). Results: Most cases (43%) were superotemporal RRD. Primary retinal reattachment was obtained in all cases, without recurrences within 3-month follow up. After surgery, a significant FAZ enlargement was observed at both the SCP and DCP level ($p < 0.001$; $p < 0.05$), with a significant effect of time noted between the two time points in the NBM and BM subanalysis ($F = 3.68$; $p < 0.017$). An excellent functional outcome was maintained for the whole follow-up. On the other hand, after surgery, perfusion parameters did not change significantly apart from the vessel density of the inferior macular sector at the DCP level ($p = 0.03$). Conclusions: Our findings suggest that the macular perfusion of eyes with RRD is still preserved if the surgery is performed really promptly, thus highlighting the great importance of a correct timing for surgery. OCTA analysis allows for a better understanding of the pathophysiological mechanisms underneath early vascular microarchitecture modifications of the posterior pole in retinal detachment, differentiating the two types of RRD not completely involving the fovea (BM and NBM).

Keywords: rhegmatogenous retinal detachment; optical coherence tomography angiography; vitrectomy; foveal avascular zone; macular vessel density

Citation: D'Aloisio, R.; Gironi, M.; Verdina, T.; Vivarelli, C.; Leonelli, R.; Mariotti, C.; Kaleci, S.; Toto, L.; Mastropasqua, R. Early Structural and Vascular Changes after Within-24 Hours Vitrectomy for Recent Onset Rhegmatogenous Retinal Detachment Treatment: A Pilot Study Comparing Bisected Macula and Not Bisected Macula. *J. Clin. Med.* **2022**, *11*, 3498. https://doi.org/10.3390/jcm11123498

Academic Editor: Andrzej Grzybowski

Received: 25 April 2022
Accepted: 11 June 2022
Published: 17 June 2022

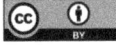

Copyright: © 2022 by the authors. Licensee MDPI, Basel, Switzerland. This article is an open access article distributed under the terms and conditions of the Creative Commons Attribution (CC BY) license (https://creativecommons.org/licenses/by/4.0/).

1. Introduction

Primary rhegmatogenous retinal detachment (RRD) is an acute threat to visual impairment due to a retinal break that allows the passage of vitreous fluid into the subretinal space. The result of this event is the separation of the neurosensory retina from the retinal pigment epithelium (RPE), requiring early surgical management [1]. Considering the morphology of the RRD, a high anatomical success rate of 82–95% has been detected following appropriate surgery [2–7]. However, the anatomical success is not always linked to functional visual recovery and involvement of the macula in the retinal detachment pathogenesis is one of the most important prognostic factors for visual prognosis [8]. In clinical practice the combination of optical coherence tomography (OCT) and optical coherence tomography angiography (OCTA) has allowed a more detailed study of some suboptimal functional recovery causes after surgery, including a refractory cystoid macular edema (CME), persistent subretinal fluid (SRF) and epiretinal membrane (ERM) combined with alteration of the inner segment/outer segment (IS/OS) [9–13], and a more accurate analysis of the pathophysiological changes occurring in the macular microcirculation in retinal diseases, such as diabetic retinopathy, age-related macular degeneration, retinal vein occlusions, uveitis and macular telangiectasias [14]. Several studies have investigated retinal microvasculature and its changes in ocular diseases after vitreoretinal surgery. Some studies based on fluorescein angiography, found a lower retinal circulation time in the detached retina and an increase in vascular resistance, leading to tissue hypoxia and to the release of inflammatory mediators [15,16]. Afterwards, some OCTA-based studies reported an enlargement of the FAZ area and a decrease in retinal vessel density, after vitrectomy, in macula-OFF RRD in comparison to eyes with Macula-ON RRD and fellow eyes [17–19]. Some prospective studies on perfusion and anatomical macular changes after surgery provided controversial results depending on surgery timing and retinal detachment features.

In this study we aimed at investigating macular perfusion/architecture modifications in eyes with early onset rhegmatogenous retinal detachment not completely involving the fovea, comparing bisected macula (BM) and not bisected macula (NBM) detachment. We aimed at highlighting the importance of a prompt surgery for visual acuity and macular perfusion status preservation, as well.

2. Materials and Methods

This study was reviewed and approved by the Local Ethics Committee of the University of Modena (Prot. AOU 0029636/20; date 20 October 2020) and Reggio Emilia and was conducted in accordance with the ethical standards of Declaration of Helsinki.

2.1. Study Subjects

In this prospective observational study, 14 eyes of 14 patients, who underwent vitreoretinal surgery for RRD, were enrolled between November 2020 and April 2021 at the Department of Ophthalmology of University of Modena and Reggio Emilia, Italy.

Only patients who successfully underwent a single uncomplicated vitreoretinal surgery for primary, recent onset (<24 h), macula-ON RRD were included. Exclusion criteria for the study were: (a) history of eye surgery within 6 previous months, (b) retinal vascular diseases, glaucoma and any other ocular diseases that may affect visual acuity or retinal/choriocapillary perfusion, (c) highly myopic eyes with axial length > 26.5 mm, (d) poor collaboration of patients during visits. All fellow eyes were healthy at the moment of data recording, and were considered as controls.

For all patients, a complete ophthalmic evaluation, including best-corrected visual acuity (BCVA, Snellen's chart, reported in LogMAR scale), slit-lamp examination, lens status (according to Lens Opacities Classification System III), applanation tonometry, axial length (AL, Aladdin TOPCON, noncontact optical low-coherence interferometry), swept source (SD)-OCT and OCTA acquisition, was performed at baseline and follow-up visits in both eyes. Postoperative data collection was set at 3 months follow-up, after complete intraocular gas reabsorption and media opacity resolutions.

Patients were further divided into two subgroups: not bisected macula group (NBM group), with retina completely attached in the area subtended by 2.5 mm diameter circle around foveola, and bisected macula group (BM group), with subretinal fluid present in that area but without causing a complete lifting. The bisected macula RD has been considered to be a macula partially involving the fovea but not completely. Extension of detachment was recorded by preoperative schematic drawing. The retina was divided into 4 quadrants of 90 degrees amplitude (superior: S, nasal: N, inferior: I, temporal: T, as reported in Table 1). A quadrant was considered involved in the detachment if it included at least 1/3 of the area.

Table 1. Demographics, ocular characteristics and surgical techniques data.

	Patients (n = 14)
Mean Age (Years)	52.6 ± 15.2
nNBM	48.13 ± 17.36
nBM	58.67 ± 10.01
Male: female (n)	8:6
RE: LE (n)	7:7
NBM	4:4
BM	3:3
PPV (SF6: C3F8) (n)	11:3
NBM: BM (n)	8:6
Diabetes mellitus [†] (n, %)	2 (14.3%)
nNBM (%)	1 (12.5%)
nBM (%)	1 (16.7%)
High blood pressure[†] (n, %)	5 (35.7%)
nNBM (%)	3 (37.5%)
nBM (%)	2 (33.3%)
Axial length (mm)	24.8 ± 1.1
nNBM	25.5 ± 1.0
nBM	24.3 ± 1.1
Phakic (n)	13
NBM: BM (n)	7:6
Pseudophakic (n)	1
NBM: BM (n)	1:0
PPV + PHACO + IOL % (n)	54.5% (6/11)
NBM: BM (n)	3:3
Surgery Duration (min)	85.36 ± 24.40
NBM	93.75 ± 24.07
BM	74.17 ± 21.78
360° laser photocoagulation % (n)	21.43% (3/14)
NBM	25% (2/8)
BM	16.67% (1/6)
Detachment extension % (n)	
S (only)	7% (1)
NBM/BM	1/0
S-N	7% (1)
NBM/BM	1/0
N (only)	0% (0)
N-I	0% (0)
I (only)	7% (1)
NBM/BM	1/0
I-T	21% (3)
NBM/BM	0/3
T (only)	14% (2)
NBM/BM	0/2
T-S	43% (6)
NBM/BM	5/1

Abbreviations: n, number of patients; RE, right eye; LE, left eye; PPV, pars plana vitrectomy; SF6, sulfur hexafluoride; C3F8 octafluoropropane; PHACO + IOL, phacoemulsification + intraocular lens implantation; BCVA, best-corrected visual acuity; S, superior; N, nasal; I, inferior; T, temporal; NBM, not bisected macula; BM, bisected macula. [†] Defined as ongoing medical treatment at the time of investigation.

2.2. OCTA Imaging

The OCT and OCTA images were acquired using Canon OCT HS100 angiography® (Canon Inc., Tokyo, Japan), whose software aims, using an appropriate algorithm, to generate a volumetric rendering of the blood flow from the internal limiting membrane (ILM) to the choroid and to allow direct visualization of the macular microcirculation. The machine performs 70,000 scans/s and the segmentation of the retinal layers is automatic and performed by the software (RX Capture for OCT-HS100®) to generate front projection images of the superficial capillary plexus (SCP) and the deep capillary plexus (DCP).

Poor-quality images (signal strength index < 8) with either significant motion artifact or extensive incorrect segmentation were excluded and repeated.

The superficial capillary plexus was analyzed considering the macular retinal section ranging from 3 μm under the ILM up to 15 μm under the internal plexiform layer (IPL). The deep capillary plexus was the thickness between 15 and 70 μm below the IPL.

Centered on the fovea, 3 × 3 mm OCTA scans were performed in both eyes. Image review was performed by two vitreoretinal specialists (R.D.A and M.G.).

The same two ophthalmologists (R.D.A. and M.G.) performed FAZ area calculation by automatically using OCTA integrated system software and by checking and manually delineating the inner edge of the foveal capillaries if errors were detected (Figure 1).

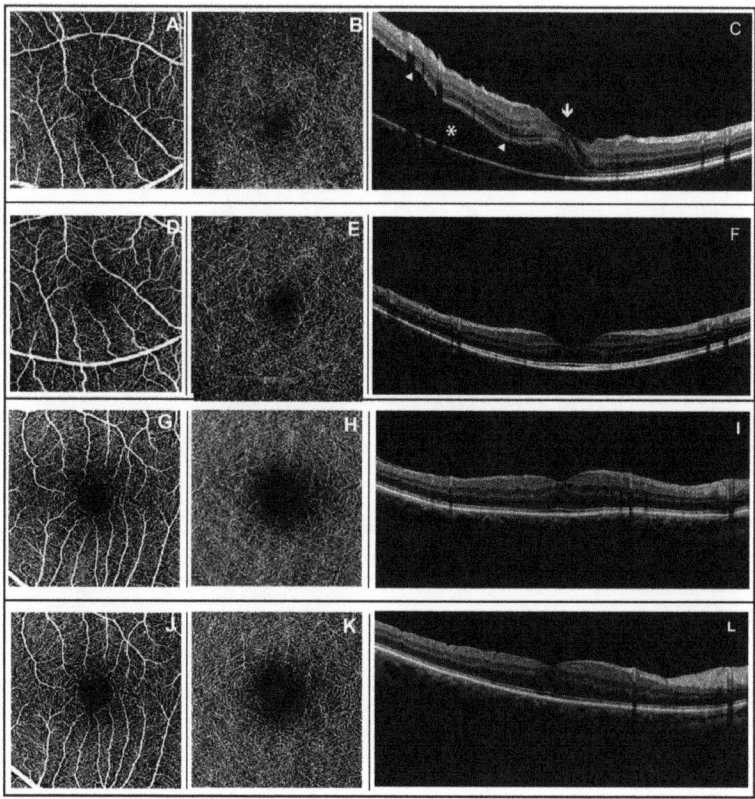

Figure 1. Foveal avascular zone area analysis on optical coherence tomography angiography en-face 3 × 3 images and optical coherence tomography B-Scan in bisected macula rhegmatogenous retinal detachment eye (**A–F**) and not bisected macula rhegmatogenous retinal detachment eye (**G–L**). (**A,G**) Superficial capillary plexus at preoperative time; (**B,H**) deep capillary plexus at preoperative time; (**C,I**) preoperative OCT B-scan of bisected and not bisected macula retinal detachment, respectively. In the bisected macula group, the subretinal fluid (*) determines a separation of the neurosensory retina (white arrowhead) from the retinal pigment epithelium that transects the fovea (white arrow), despite that, the fovea remains morphologically intact. (**D,J**) Superficial capillary plexus at postoperative time; (**E,K**) deep capillary plexus at postoperative time; (**F,L**) postoperative OCT B-scan of bisected and not bisected macula retinal detachment. In the bisected macula group, restoration of normal morphology has occurred following retinal detachment repair.

VD and vessel length density (VLD) were recorded for central area (fVD/fVLD, the area under a circumference of 1 mm diameter around the fovea), parafoveal area (pfVD/pfVLD, annular area extending between 1 and 2.5 mm diameter, centered on the foveola) and whole macular area (wVD/wVLD, area under a circumference of 2.5 mm diameter around the fovea). In addition, parafoveal area was segmented in four quadrants (superior, nasal, inferior and temporal), then VD and VLD were recorded for each of them. All these processes of segmentation of macular OCTA images were performed by integrated images processing system software (Figure 2).

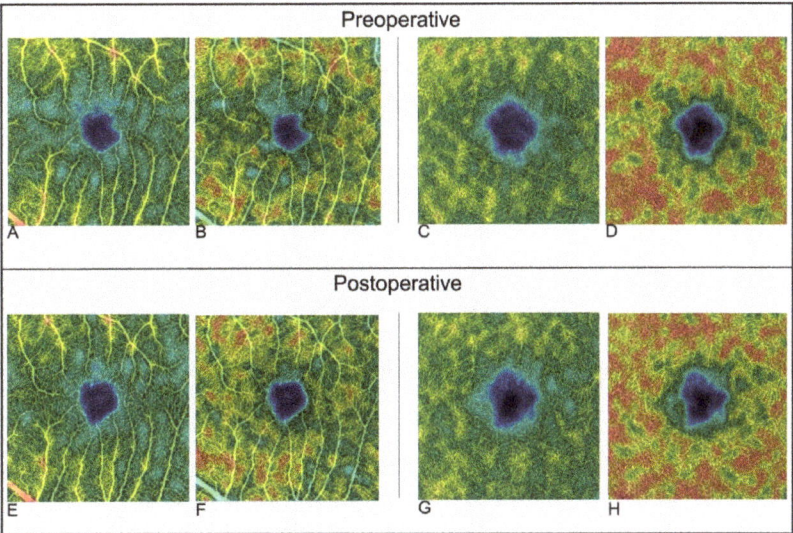

Figure 2. Optical coherence tomography angiography 3 × 3 density map images in macula ON rhegmatogenous retinal detachment eyes. Preoperative vessel density and vessel length density of superficial capillary plexus (**A**,**B**); vessel density and vessel length density of deep capillary plexus at preoperative time (**C**,**D**). Postoperative vessel density and vessel length density of superficial capillary plexus (**E**,**F**); Postoperative vessel density and vessel length density of deep capillary plexus (**G**,**H**).

VD and VLD values were calculated, automatically, by the same integrated system, for each plexus.

In order to calculate VD, the software (OCT-HS100 Angio Expert AX®) creates a binary image from an OCTA image and indicates the percentage of white pixels in the region by percent (%). Then, for the calculation of VLD (skeletonization of the image), it transforms the lines of a binary image, created from an OCTA image, into thin lines (1 pixel of thickness) and indicates the value obtained by dividing the sum of the length of the thin lines in the region by the area by "mm^{-1}". CMT was calculated using retinal thickness map of SS-OCT, in Macula 3D mode. In the case of BM group RRDs, manual editing of the retinal thickness boundary lines was performed to calculate the CMT value.

2.3. Surgical Procedure

All surgical procedures were performed by the same expert vitreoretinal surgeon (R.M.) within 24 hours. All patients were treated with 25 gauge-pars plana vitrectomy, with diluted gas as tamponade (SF6 (20%) or C3F8 (12%)), with final expansible gas injection.

In all cases, standard three-port-PPV was performed with Stellaris vitrectomy machine (Bausch & Lomb Incorporated, Rochester, NY, USA). Central and peripheral vitrectomy was performed, followed by fluid-air exchange and laser retinopexy. Combined cataract surgery was performed in phakic eyes depending on lens status.

2.4. Statistical Analysis

Statistical analysis was performed with STATA® software version 14 (StataCorp. 2015. Stata Statistical Software: Release 14. College Station, TX, USA: StataCorp LP). The main outcome parameters included the percentage of BM vs. NBM, and BCVA, CMT, FAZ area of SCP and DCP, VD and VLD of SCP and DCP, expressed as mean ± SD. The normality of the sample distribution was confirmed using the Shapiro–Wilk test ($p > 0.05$). Statistical differences for continuous variable for two groups were examined using paired and unpaired Student's t test. The homogeneity of variances was calculated by Levene Test. The One-Way ANOVA test was used, with post hoc Bonferroni test, to analyze the measurements in each area. Correlation analysis between the values in the different locations were investigated by Pearson's correlation test. Margins are statistic calculated from predictions of a previously fit model at fixed values of some covariates and averaging. The margins estimate the margins of responses for specified values of covariates and present the results as a figure.

2.5. Box Plot Analysis

Box plots were used to visualize differences in the distribution of numerical data between different groups. The differences between two groups were analyzed by calculating the fold change and p-value (Student's t-test).

2.6. Scatter Plot Analysis

Scatter plots were used to display relationships between two numeric variables, and the strength and direction of the linear relationships were assessed by Pearson's correlation coefficient. A $p < 0.05$ was considered statistically significant. p-value ≤ 0.05 was considered of statistical significance.

3. Results

A total of 14 eyes of 14 patients (eight men, six women) with a mean age of 52.6 ± 15.2 years old were included in this study between November 2020 and April 2021. All patients had a macula ON RRD (six RRD with bisected macula, BM group; eight with not bisected macula, NBM group). The fellow eyes were considered as controls. Patients' baseline demographic parameters, ocular characteristics and surgical information are summarized in Table 1.

Primary retinal reattachment was obtained in all cases, without recurrences within 3-month follow up. PPV with C3F8 (12%) tamponade was performed in three eyes, while SF6 (20%) was used in 11 eyes. No intraoperative and postoperative complications were observed. None of the eyes included in our study showed extension retinal detachment involving more than two quadrants (Table 1). The retinal detachment mainly involved the superior and temporal sectors (temporal: 78%; superior: 57%; inferior: 28%; nasal: 7%; Table 1).

3.1. OCTA Findings

Overall, the mean FAZ area in the affected eyes showed a significant enlargement postsurgery compared to preoperative values, both in the SCP and DCP ($p = 0.0003$ and $p = 0.0107$, respectively) (Table 2).

Table 2. Best-corrected visual acuity, optical coherence tomography and optical coherence tomography angiography mean values.

	Preoperative	Postoperative	Fellow Eye	p-Value Pre. vs. Post.	p-Value Pre. vs. Fellow
BCVA (logMAR)	0.114 ± 0.2	0.089 ± 0.184	0.016 ± 0.059	0.3644	0.1144
(Snellen)	20/26	20/25	20/20		
CMT (μm)	307.50 ± 35.56	302.64 ± 33.84	284.64 ± 26.47	0.5914	**0.0067**
FAZ (mm2)					
Scp	0.24 ± 0.08	0.33 ± 0.13	0.24 ± 0.09	**0.0003**	0.8739
Dcp	0.35 ± 0.16	0.45 ± 0.24	0.36 ± 0.15	**0.0107**	0.0941
Central Area					
VD (%) Scp	32.24 ± 4.55	29.54 ± 4.79	30.62 ± 4.35	0.1298	0.0758
VD (%) Dcp	32.63 ± 9.81	30.70 ± 6.77	29.63 ± 6.83	0.4378	0.1486
VLD (mm^{-1}) Scp	18.22 ± 3.11	16.29 ± 2.72	17.6 ± 2.60	0.1074	0.3980
VLD (mm^{-1}) Dcp	19.67 ± 6.35	18.44 ± 4.27	17.77 ± 4.86	0.4443	0.1773
Quadrant I					
VD (%) Scp	41.58 ± 3.93	42.01 ± 2.15	42.06 ± 3.45	0.6224	0.7051
VD (%) Dcp	42.72 ± 3.69	44.1 ± 2.42	43.96 ± 3.4	**0.0357**	0.2991
VLD (mm^{-1}) Scp	22.94 ± 3.15	22.07 ± 2.89	22.99 ± 3.25	0.2841	0.9500
VLD (mm^{-1}) Dcp	26.82 ± 3.12	26.91 ± 2.76	26.47 ± 3.19	0.9294	0.6561
Quadrant N					
VD (%) Scp	37.3 ± 7.07	37.34 ± 3.77	39.27 ± 2.42	0.9838	0.3395
VD (%) Dcp	41.51 ± 4.16	41.03 ± 3.70	43.06 ± 2.44	0.7448	0.1063
VLD (mm^{-1}) Scp	21.13 ± 4.89	20.54 ± 3.55	21.95 ± 2.73	0.6137	0.4177
VLD (mm^{-1}) Dcp	25.63 ± 3.26	25.19 ± 2.77	26.28 ± 2.36	0.6562	0.3093
Quadrant S					
VD (%) Scp	41.29 ± 3.90	39.04 ± 4.76	42.84 ± 2.15	0.1884	0.2025
VD (%) Dcp	44.59 ± 2.68	41.88 ± 5.2	43.67 ± 2.53	0.0748	0.1279
VLD (mm^{-1}) Scp	22.74 ± 3.22	20.91 ± 3.92	23.34 ± 3.28	0.0779	0.2915
VLD (mm^{-1}) Dcp	27.93 ± 2.92	25.84 ± 4.27	26.79 ± 3.56	0.1959	0.2436
Quadrant T					
VD (%) Scp	40.34 ± 4.13	37.78 ± 2.72	40.3 ± 1.78	0.0749	0.9774
VD (%) Dcp	42.96 ± 2.96	42.24 ± 2.3	42.75 ± 1.57	0.4299	0.8184
VLD (mm^{-1}) Scp	22.41 ± 2.78	20.69 ± 2.95	22.29 ± 2.47	0.1130	0.8921
VLD (mm^{-1}) Dcp	26.68 ± 2.75	25.91 ± 3.05	25.89 ± 2.65	0.5471	0.3824
Whole Macular Area					
VD (%) Scp	38.55 ± 3.50	37.14 ± 2.88	39.02 ± 2.10	0.2855	0.5915
VD (%) Dcp	40.89 ± 4.00	39.99 ± 3.47	40.61 ± 2.92	0.3868	0.7796
VLD (mm^{-1}) Scp	21.49 ± 2.72	20.1 ± 2.88	21.63 ± 2.50	0.0980	0.7796
VLD (mm^{-1}) Dcp	25.35 ± 2.76	24.46 ± 2.85	24.64 ± 2.98	0.3633	0.2758
Parafoveal Macular Area					
VD (%) Scp	40.13 ± 3.82	39.04 ± 2.88	41.12 ± 1.81	0.3981	0.3580
VD (%) Dcp	42.94 ± 2.77	42.31 ± 2.91	43.36 ± 2.11	0.4068	0.5140
VLD (mm^{-1}) Scp	22.31 ± 2.92	21.05 ± 3.19	22.64 ± 2.70	0.1231	0.5150
VLD (mm^{-1}) Dcp	26.76 ± 2.55	25.97 ± 2.89	26.36 ± 2.80	0.4472	0.5205

BCVA: Best-corrected visual acuity; CMT: central macular thickness; FAZ: foveal avascular zone; VD: vessel density; VLD: vessel length density; SCP: superficial capillary plexus; DCP: deep capillary plexus.

In a subanalysis between the BM and NBM subgroups, postoperative SCP FAZ enlargement was significant in both groups (Table 3). In detail, for the BM group postoperative SCP FAZ (mean 0.35 ± 0.15 mm^2) was significantly ($p < 0.05$) improved compared with the preoperative (mean 0.24 ± 0.09 mm^2) and the fellow group (mean 0.25 ± 0.11 mm^2). The postoperative SCP FAZ (mean 0.31 ± 0.12 mm^2) was the largest ($p < 0.05$) compared with the preoperative (mean 0.24 ± 0.08 mm^2) in NBM group. No significant difference was observed between the preoperative and fellow group in the BM and NBM groups (Table 3).

Table 3. Best-corrected visual acuity and optical coherence tomography angiography mean values for the BM and NBM groups.

	BM			NBM		
	Preoperative	Postoperative	Fellow Eye	Preoperative	Postoperative	Fellow Eye
BCVA (logMAR)	0.24 ± 0.26	0.16 ± 0.27	0.04 ± 0.08	0.01 ± 0.03 [#]	0.03 ± 0.03	0.0 ± 0.0
FAZ (mm^2)						
Scp	0.24 ± 0.09	0.35 ± 0.15 *	0.25 ± 0.11	0.24 ± 0.08	0.31 ± 0.12 °	0.23 ± 0.07
Dcp	0.32 ± 0.18	0.42 ± 0.29 *	0.34 ± 0.16	0.36 ± 0.14	0.46 ± 0.22	0.37 ± 0.15
Whole Macular Area						
VD (%) Scp	40.21 ± 3.19	36.67 ± 3.43	38.49 ± 2.21	37.30 ± 3.36	37.49 ± 2.58	39.41 ± 2.05
VD (%) Dcp	42.03 ± 3.78	40.26 ± 2.51	40.52 ± 3.38	40.02 ± 4.17	39.78 ± 4.20	40.67 ± 2.76
VLD (mm^{-1}) Scp	23.23 ± 1.62	20.66 ± 2.84	22.25 ± 1.66	20.18 ± 2.70	19.67 ± 3.01	21.16 ± 3.01
VLD (mm^{-1}) Dcp	26.81 ± 2.46	25.14 ± 0.89	25.64 ± 1.40	24.24 ± 2.56	23.95 ± 3.72	23.88 ± 2.63

* Statistically significant, p-value < 0.05 for Faz in BM group, pre vs. post; ° statistically significant, p-value < 0.05 for Faz in NBM group, pre vs. post; [#] statistically significant, p-value < 0.05 for BCVA in preoperative group, BM vs. NBM.

Conversely, postoperative DCP FAZ significantly increased only in the BM subgroup (Table 3).

A significant effect of time was also noted between the two time points (F = 3.68; $p < 0.017$) for FAZ between BM and NBM (Figure 3).

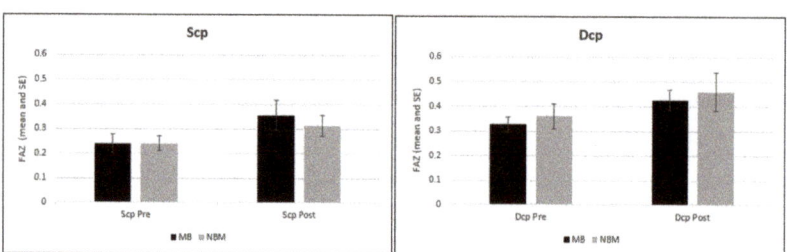

Figure 3. Estimated marginal means preoperative and postoperative described for each DCP and SCP plexuses for the BM and NBM groups.

No statistically significant correlations were found between BCVA and FAZ in either the SCP ($p = 0.50$) or DCP ($p = 0.14$). No significant correlations were found between the final BCVA and CMT ($p = 0.43$). An inverse correlation was found between the SCP FAZ and the CMT ($p = 0.0078$) but not for the DCP FAZ ($p = 0.088$).

Regarding perfusion parameters, a decreasing trend was observed in terms of whole macular VD in both the DCP and SCP after surgery. In detail, the quantitative analysis of the individual quadrants showed a trend of decreased perfusion in all sectors except for the nasal one, but not significantly, and the inferior one, which was found to be statistically significant higher in the DCP ($p = 0.036$, Figure 4) and slightly increased in the SCP layer.

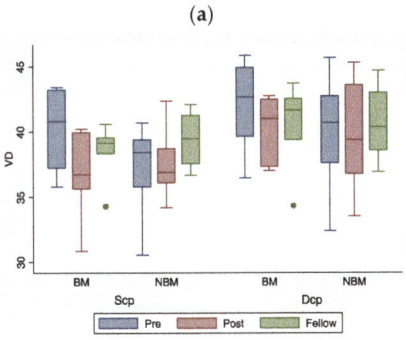 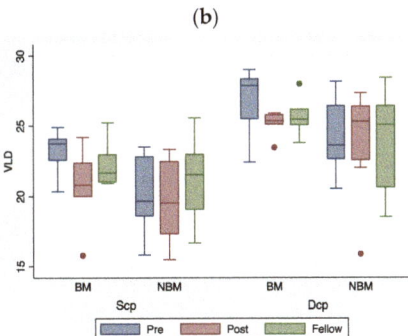

Figure 4. Boxplot showing distribution of VD (**a**) and VLD (**b**) in both DCP and SCP after, before surgery and fellow eye results for the BM and NBM groups. Boxes represent interquartile range, whiskers represent variability and horizontal bars represent the median value.

An inverse trend between the mean FAZ area, and the values of fVD and fVLD were found both in the SCP and DCP. No correlation was found between the perfusion parameters and final visual outcomes, in both plexuses.

No correlation between the surgery time and postoperative SCP FAZ (p = 0.59), DCP FAZ (p = 0.69) and CMT (p = 0.72) was assessed.

3.2. Visual Acuity

No difference in terms of visual acuity was found between RRD eyes and the fellow ones (Table 2). In diseased eyes, the mean BCVA was 0.11 ± 0.20 logMAR and 0.089 ± 0.180 logMAR preoperatively and postoperatively, respectively, without statistical differences (Table 2). The choice of the tamponade gas or the entity of laser photocoagulation (360° or sectorial) had no statistically significant effect on the final visual outcome.

4. Discussion

In this prospective observational study, our sample showed changes in retinal architecture and vascularization in patients with early onset macula-ON RRD treated with prompt vitreoretinal surgery (within 24 hours). These early anatomical and perfusion modifications were analyzed using OCTA, which nowadays has become a clinical practice tool able of rapidly and non-invasively assessing macular perfusion and architecture.

At baseline, no significant difference was found between eyes with RRD and fellow eyes in terms of FAZ area, thus suggesting that probably more time is required for anatomical microstructural changes to occur in early onset macula on RRD and that surgery itself may be partially responsible for the structural modification. Indeed, similarly to previous studies, our findings described a statistically significant enlargement of the FAZ area postoperatively, in comparison to preoperative values, in both of the two retinal capillary plexuses (SCP and DCP), as an indirect sign of ischemic changes or retinal manipulation during surgery [17–19].

Of note, in our subanalysis between BM and NBM subgroups, postoperative SCP FAZ enlargement was significant in both BM and NBM, while postoperative DCP FAZ enlargement was significant only in the BM subgroup. The maintenance of the foveal microstructure has been strictly linked to the postsurgical visual outcome in macula off retinal detachment. Our data, based on a relatively short follow-up time, reported an excellent visual outcome preservation, given that the macula was not or only partially involved. Nevertheless, in the macula ON RRD condition, some previous works did not report any significant difference between pre and postoperative FAZ values in the eyes of patients who underwent vitreoretinal surgery [17,20–24]. Barca et al. observed a reduction, not statistically significant, in the FAZ area of operated eyes, but this could probably be explained by peeling of the ILM, performed for all patients in the study, which could be responsible for a decrease in and/or distortion of the FAZ area [24,25]. Barca et al. also reported that eyes with macula ON RRD showed significant preoperative lowering of VD when compared with fellow eyes at the SCP level, recovering over time after 6 month follow-up [20,21,24]. The authors explained the phenomenon assuming that peripheral retinal vascular resistance during RRD could induce a detectable slowing of blood perfusion in the SCP. Previous studies on eyes with macula OFF RRD, using fluorescein angiography, had already identified how increased vascular resistance in the detached retina could lead to a reduction in and slowing of blood flow [15,16,26,27]. By means of scanning laser Doppler flowmetry, Eshita T. et al. reported the mechanical effect of scleral buckle indentation on peripheral perfusion, which caused a blood flow decrease just two weeks after surgery in patients with RRD without macular involvement; nevertheless, a complete reperfusion was observed after 1-month follow up, reaching baseline values [27]. Chua et al., in a prospective study reporting 1-year follow-up findings, observed a FAZ area decrease, explained as a likely physiological variability in the FAZ size; nevertheless, they considered only macula OFF RRD patients [28].

Conversely, in our cohort of patients with RRD, at baseline, whole macular and parafoveal VD and VLD of diseased eyes were slightly decreased when compared with the fellow ones, but not significantly. After surgery, the whole macular and parafoveal VD and VLD of our sample had a downward trend in both retinal plexuses. In detail, we noticed a slight decrease in VD and VLD in all retinal layers analyzed (SCP and DCP) and a statistical rise in VD at the deep level of the inferior quadrants of the posterior pole, likely due to the main topographical involvement of retinal detachment in our cohort of patients (43% superotemporal involvement). Yi et al. found that, in the case of hypoxia, an abnormal oxygen metabolism could increase the metabolic demands of the retinal circulation, rather than increasing the extraction of oxygen from the choriocapillaris. Therefore, in the case of RRD, hypoxia would occur in the detached retina with a consequent increased oxygen extraction starting from the retinal vascularization [29]. Moreover, blood flow changes after surgery have been significantly correlated with the extent of RRD [27].

Our findings partially agree with previous publications, where they did not report any changes in VD after vitreoretinal surgery [17,20–23]. Obviously, it should be taken into consideration that a part of our sample consisted of eyes with macula bisected solved within 24 hours from the onset of symptoms, allowing us to speculate that the retinal perfusion might start to behave as a macula off retinal detachment unless an immediate surgical correction is performed. We may further hypothesize that the retina attached immediately adjacent to the detached retina is more sensitive to hypoxic damage related to slowing blood flow. Despite the retinal flow decreased in retinal detachment pathogenesis, we may assume that this was not sufficiently low or more time was needed from the onset of the retinal detachment to induce microstructural changes detectable with OCTA on the whole macular area in our study population.

Similarly to our results, Yoshikawa et al. reported no significant difference in macular perfusion density between eyes with retinal detachment and the healthy fellow eyes, underlining that early onset retinal detachment keeps the retinal vasculature intact. Differently to this, Bonfiglio et al. focused their attention on a retrospective cohort of patients with an anatomically attached retina after at least 12 months from surgery, dividing them into two subgroups, macula on and off. In the macula on group, no significant difference in postoperative mean FMT, FAZ and SCP VD was found, while a lower mean DCP VD in the parafoveal subfield was assessed. It is still debated as to which capillary plexus is first involved in retinal detachment. Woo et al. hypothesized that the DCP is more vulnerable to a lack of oxygen because of its different anatomical vascular supply and different intraretinal location compared with the SCP, which is directly connected to the retinal arterioles instead of the venous channels. Conversely, other works found that in early onset retinal detachment, especially when the macula is spared, the most affected capillary plexus seems to be the SCP, which is the first vascular layer involved in a fast increase in vascular resistance induced by the RRD. The SCP may develop a stronger and faster contraction than the DCP due to its greater density of arterioles and smooth muscle. Conversely, the DCP, although more vulnerable to damage caused by hypoxia, could be involved later [24].

Moreover, in the retinal detachment pathophysiology, Muller cells seem to be another important factor in the mechanisms of vasoconstriction and hypoxia. Activated by the release of Endothelin-1, they can cause alterations in the internal retinal flow, even in the absence of structural alterations [30–32]. In addition, Endothelin-1, which was found to be increased in the subretinal fluid in RRD eyes, has an intrinsic vasoconstrictive action, leading to a reduction in microvascular blood flow [33,34]. Unfortunately, we did not analyze Endothelin-1 or other cytokines' levels in subretinal fluid.

The unique angle of this prospective work was the analysis of early microvascular and microarchitectural alterations in patients with early onset macula ON retinal detachment who underwent prompt vitreoretinal surgery within 24 hours, thus suggesting a predictive role of such perfusion changes as potential biomarkers of final prognosis after surgery and underlining the importance of a correct timing in macula ON DRR surgery. A subanalysis between bisected and not bisected macula was reported as well, adding a new understanding into the field.

It is still controversial if macular vessel changes could actually be related to visual prognosis. In our study, no statistically significant differences were identified in terms of mean BCVA either between preoperative and postoperative values. This is important given that our study involved only patients with macula ON RRD. In the literature, macular involvement is one of the main factors influencing postoperative visual acuity, especially in relation to the duration of detachment [35,36]. As expected, our sample showed a worse visual acuity in BM patients in comparison with the NBM group. Despite this, no significant differences in final postsurgical BCVA were detected between the two subgroups. This is in accordance with previous studies, where the progression of detachment to macular involvement does not consistently influence visual functional recovery if surgery is performed very quickly (within 24 hours) [26,37,38]. No significant correlation was found between BCVA and FAZ in both the SCP and DCP as well.

In addition to this, in our sample, the inverse relationship between FAZ and CMT was respected as previously reported in several studies, both in healthy and RRD macula ON eyes [15,22,24,39].

5. Conclusions

In conclusion, our findings suggest that BM and NBM groups could behave differently in terms of structural parameters such as FAZ. On the other hand, macular perfusion of eyes with macula-on RRD, also with the macula not yet completely involved as in the bisected one, is still preserved if the surgery is performed promptly; thus highlighting the great importance of a correct timing for surgery, in both cases of BM and NBM.

Undoubtedly, our study has some limitations. First, the sample size of the study group was relatively small with a relatively short follow-up period of 3 months. Second, some surgical parameters that could influence the recovery of the capillary plexuses such as the elevation of IOP during surgery were not considered in our study. Third, vitreous or SRF chemokine/cytokines levels to be correlated with perfusion/architectural parameters were not investigated.

Further investigations are needed with a wider sample of patients, with a longer follow-up period and with a correlation between perfusion parameters and the extent of detached retina, to better understand the pathophysiological mechanism underneath these early vascular microarchitecture modifications of the posterior pole in retinal detachment not completely involving the fovea. A prospective longer study would be warranted to confirm and validate this preliminary results.

Author Contributions: Conceptualization, R.M.; methodology, C.M.; formal analysis, S.K.; investigation, T.V. and C.V.; data curation, R.L.; writing—original draft preparation, M.G. and L.T.; writing—review and editing, R.D. and R.M.; supervision, C.M. All authors have read and agreed to the published version of the manuscript.

Funding: This research received no external funding.

Institutional Review Board Statement: This study was reviewed and approved by the Local Ethics Committee of the University of Modena (Prot. AOU 0029636/20; date 20 October 2020) and Reggio Emilia.

Informed Consent Statement: Informed consent was obtained from all subjects involved in the study.

Data Availability Statement: All data will be available on request to the corresponding author.

Conflicts of Interest: The authors declare no conflict of interest.

References

1. Kuhn, F.; Aylward, B. Rhegmatogenous retinal detachment: A reappraisal of its pathophysiology and treatment. *Ophthalmic Res.* **2014**, *51*, 15–31. [CrossRef]
2. Nemet, A.; Moshiri, A.; Yiu, G.; Loewenstein, A.; Moisseiev, E. A Review of Innovations in Rhegmatogenous Retinal Detachment Surgical Techniques. *J. Ophthalmol.* **2017**, *2017*, 4310643. [CrossRef] [PubMed]
3. Thompson, J.A.; Snead, M.P.; Billington, B.M.; Barrie, T.; Thompson, J.R.; Sparrow, J.M. National audit of the outcome of primary surgery for rhegmatogenous retinal detachment. II. Clinical outcomes. *Eye* **2002**, *16*, 771–777. [CrossRef]
4. Dhoot, A.S.; Popovic, M.M.; Nichani, P.A.H.; Eshtiaghi, A.; Mihalache, A.; Sayal, A.P.; Yu, H.; Wykoff, C.C.; Kertes, P.J.; Muni, R.H. Pars plana vitrectomy versus scleral buckle: A comprehensive meta-analysis of 15,947 eyes. *Surv. Ophthalmol.* **2022**, *67*, 932–949. [CrossRef] [PubMed]
5. Kobashi, H.; Takano, M.; Yanagita, T.; Shiratani, T.; Wang, G.; Hoshi, K.; Shimizu, K. Scleral buckling and pars plana vitrectomy for rhegmatogenous retinal detachment: An analysis of 542 eyes. *Curr. Eye Res.* **2014**, *39*, 204–211. [CrossRef] [PubMed]
6. Orlin, A.; Hewing, N.J.; Nissen, M.; Lee, S.; Kiss, S.; D'Amico, D.J.; Chan, R.V.P. Pars plana vitrectomy compared with pars plana vitrectomy combined with scleral buckle in the primary management of noncomplex rhegmatogenous retinal detachment. *Retina* **2014**, *34*, 1069–1075. [CrossRef]
7. Lumi, X.; Lužnik, Z.; Petrovski, G.; Petrovski, B.É.; Hawlina, M. Anatomical success rate of pars plana vitrectomy for treatment of complex rhegmatogenous retinal detachment. *BMC Ophthalmol.* **2016**, *16*, 216. [CrossRef]
8. van Bussel, E.M.; van der Valk, R.; Bijlsma, W.R.; La Heij, E.C. Impact of duration of macula-off retinal detachment on visual outcome: A systematic review and meta-analysis of literature. *Retina* **2014**, *34*, 1917–1925. [CrossRef]
9. Tee, J.J.L.; Veckeneer, M.; Laidlaw, D.A. Persistent subfoveolar fluid following retinal detachment surgery: An SD-OCT guided study on the incidence, aetiological associations, and natural history. *Eye* **2016**, *30*, 481–487. [CrossRef]
10. Ghassemi, F.; Karkhaneh, R.; Rezaei, M.; Nili-Ahmadabadi, M.; Ebrahimiadib, N.; Roohipoor, R.; Mohammadi, N. Foveal structure in macula-off rhegmatogenous retinal detachment after scleral buckling or vitrectomy. *J. Ophthalmic Vis. Res.* **2015**, *10*, 172–177. [CrossRef]
11. Karacorlu, M.; Muslubas, I.S.; Hocaoglu, M.; Arf, S.; Ersoz, M.G. Correlation between morphological changes and functional outcomes of recent-onset macula-off rhegmatogenous retinal detachment: Prognostic factors in rhegmatogenous retinal detachment. *Int. Ophthalmol.* **2018**, *38*, 1275–1283. [CrossRef] [PubMed]
12. Kang, H.M.; Lee, S.C.; Lee, C.S. Association of Spectral-Domain Optical Coherence Tomography Findings with Visual Outcome of Macula-Off Rhegmatogenous Retinal Detachment Surgery. *Ophthalmologica* **2015**, *234*, 83–90. [CrossRef] [PubMed]
13. Poulsen, C.D.; Petersen, M.P.; Green, A.; Peto, T.; Grauslund, J. Fundus autofluorescence and spectral domain optical coherence tomography as predictors for long-term functional outcome in rhegmatogenous retinal detachment. *Graefe's Arch. Clin. Exp. Ophthalmol.* **2019**, *257*, 715–723. [CrossRef]
14. Agrawal, R.; Xin, W.; Keane, P.A.; Chhablani, J.; Agarwal, A. Optical coherence tomography angiography: A non-invasive tool to image end-arterial system. *Expert Rev. Med Devices* **2016**, *13*, 519–521. [CrossRef]
15. Satoh, Y. Retinal circulation in rhegmatogenous retinal detachment demonstrated by videofluorescence angiography and image analysis. I. The condition of retinal circulation before retinal detachment surgery. *Nippon Ganka Gakkai Zasshi (Acta Soc. Ophthalmol. Jpn.)* **1989**, *93*, 1002–1008.
16. Piccolino, C.; Piccolino, F. Vascular Changes in Rhegmatogenous Retinal Detachment. *Ophthalmologica* **1983**, *186*, 17–24. [CrossRef]
17. Woo, J.E.; Yoon, Y.S.; Min, J.K. Foveal Avascular Zone Area Changes Analyzed Using OCT Angiography after Successful Rhegmatogenous Retinal Detachment Repair. *Curr. Eye Res.* **2018**, *43*, 674–678. [CrossRef]
18. Sato, T.; Kanai, M.; Busch, C.; Wakabayashi, T. Foveal avascular zone area after macula-off rhegmatogenous retinal detachment repair: An optical coherence tomography angiography study. *Graefe's Arch. Clin. Exp. Ophthalmol.* **2017**, *255*, 2071–2072. [CrossRef] [PubMed]

19. Agarwal, A.; Aggarwal, K.; Akella, M.; Agrawal, R.; Khandelwal, N.; Bansal, R.; Singh, R.; Gupta, V. Fractal Dimension and Optical Coherence Tomography Angiography Features of the Central Macula After Repair of Rhegmatogenous Rental Detachmnets. *Retina* **2019**, *39*, 2167–2177. [CrossRef]
20. Yoshikawa, Y.; Shoji, T.; Kanno, J.; Ibuki, H.; Ozaki, K.; Ishii, H.; Ichikawa, Y.; Kimura, I.; Shinoda, K. Evaluation of microvascular changes in the macular area of eyes with rhegmatogenous retinal detachment without macular involvement using swept-source optical coherence tomography angiography. *Clin. Ophthalmol.* **2018**, *12*, 2059–2067. [CrossRef]
21. Chatziralli, I.; Theodossiadis, G.; Parikakis, E.; Chatzirallis, A.; Dimitriou, E.; Theodossiadis, P. Inner retinal layers' alterations and microvasculature changes after vitrectomy for rhegmatogenous retinal detachment. *Int. Ophthalmol.* **2020**, *40*, 3349–3356. [CrossRef] [PubMed]
22. Bonfiglio, V.; Ortisi, E.; Scollo, D.; Reibaldi, M.; Russo, A.; Pizzo, A.; Faro, G.; Macchi, I.; Fallico, M.; Toro, M.D.; et al. Vascular changes after vitrectomy for rhegmatogenous retinal detachment: Optical coherence tomography angiography study. *Acta Ophthalmol.* **2019**, *98*, 563. [CrossRef] [PubMed]
23. Hong, E.H.; Cho, H.; Kim, D.R.; Kang, M.H.; Shin, Y.U.; Seong, M. Changes in Retinal Vessel and Retinal Layer Thickness After Vitrectomy in Retinal Detachment via Swept-Source OCT Angiography. *Investig. Opthalmol. Vis. Sci.* **2020**, *61*, 35. [CrossRef] [PubMed]
24. Barca, F.; Bacherini, D.; Dragotto, F.; Tartaro, R.; Lenzetti, C.; Finocchio, L.; Rizzo, S.; Savastano, A.; Giansanti, F.; Caporossi, T.; et al. OCT Angiography Findings in Macula-ON and Macula-OFF Rhegmatogenous Retinal Detachment: A Prospective Study. *J. Clin. Med.* **2020**, *9*, 3982. [CrossRef]
25. Baba, T.; Kakisu, M.; Nizawa, T.; Oshitari, T.; Yamamoto, S. Study of foveal avascular zone by OCTA before and after idiopathic epiretinal membrane removal. *Spektrum Augenheilkd.* **2017**, *32*, 31–38. [CrossRef]
26. Lee, C.S.; Shaver, K.; Yun, S.H.; Kim, D.; Wen, S.; Ghorayeb, G. Comparison of the visual outcome between macula-on and macula-off rhegmatogenous retinal detachment based on the duration of macular detachment. *BMJ Open Ophthalmol.* **2021**, *6*, e000615. [CrossRef] [PubMed]
27. Eshita, T.; Shinoda, K.; Kimura, I.; Kitamura, S.; Ishida, S.; Inoue, M.; Mashima, Y.; Katsura, H.; Oguchi, Y. Retinal Blood Flow in the Macular Area Before and After Scleral Buckling Procedures for Rhegmatogenous Retinal Detachment Without Macular Involvement. *Jpn. J. Ophthalmol.* **2004**, *48*, 358–363. [CrossRef]
28. Chua, J.; Ke, M.; Tan, B.; Gan, A.T.L.; Lim, L.S.; Tan, G.S.; Lee, S.Y.; Wong, E.; Schmetterer, L.; Cheung, N. Association of macular and choroidal perfusion with long-term visual outcomes after macula-off rhegmatogenous retinal detachmen. *Br. J. Ophthalmol.* **2021**. [CrossRef]
29. Yi, J.; Liu, W.; Chen, S.; Backman, V.; Sheibani, N.; Sorenson, C.M.; Fawzi, A.A.; Linsenmeier, R.A.; Zhang, H.F. Visible light optical coherence tomography measures retinal oxygen metabolic response to systemic oxygenation. *Light. Sci. Appl.* **2015**, *4*, e334. [CrossRef]
30. Iandiev, I.; Uhlmann, S.; Pietsch, U.-C.; Biedermann, B.; Reichenbach, A.; Wiedemann, P.; Bringmann, A. Endothelin receptors in the detached retina of the pig. *Neurosci. Lett.* **2005**, *384*, 72–75. [CrossRef]
31. Iandiev, I. Glial Cell Reactivity in a Porcine Model of Retinal Detachment. *Investig. Opthalmol. Vis. Sci.* **2006**, *47*, 2161–2171. [CrossRef] [PubMed]
32. Gaucher, D.; Chiappore, J.-A.; Pâques, M.; Simonutti, M.; Boitard, C.; Sahel, J.A.; Massin, P.; Picaud, S. Microglial changes occur without neural cell death in diabetic retinopathy. *Vis. Res.* **2007**, *47*, 612–623. [CrossRef] [PubMed]
33. Roldán-Pallarés, M.; Musa, A.-S.; Hernández-Montero, J.; Llatas, C.B. Preoperative duration of retinal detachment and preoperative central retinal artery hemodynamics: Repercussion on visual acuity. *Graefe's Arch. Clin. Exp. Ophthalmol.* **2009**, *247*, 625–631. [CrossRef]
34. Polak, K.; Luksch, A.; Frank, B.; Jandrasits, K.; Polska, E.; Schmetterer, L. Regulation of human retinal blood low by endothelin-1. *Exp. Eye Res.* **2003**, *76*, 633–640. [CrossRef]
35. Williamson, T.H.; Shunmugam, M.; Rodrigues, I.; Dogramaci, M.; Lee, E. Characteristics of rhegmatogenous retinal detachment and their relationship to visual outcome. *Eye* **2013**, *27*, 1063–1069. [CrossRef] [PubMed]
36. Salicone, A.; Smiddy, W.E.; Venkatraman, A.; Feuer, W. Visual recovery after scleral buckling procedure for retinal detachment. *Ophthalmology* **2006**, *113*, 1734–1742. [CrossRef] [PubMed]
37. Kontos, A.; Williamson, T.H. Rate and risk factors for the conversion of fovea-on to fovea-off rhegmatogenous retinal detachment while awaiting surgery. *Br. J. Ophthalmol.* **2017**, *101*, 1011–1015. [CrossRef]
38. Angermann, R.; Bechrakis, N.E.; Rauchegger, T.; Casazza, M.; Nowosielski, Y.; Zehetner, C. Effect of Timing on Visual Outcomes in Fovea-Involving Retinal Detachments Verified by SD-OCT. *J. Ophthalmol.* **2020**, *2020*, 2307935. [CrossRef]
39. Samara, W.A.; Say, E.A.T.; Khoo, C.T.L.; Higgins, T.P.; Magrath, G.; Ferenczy, S.; Shields, C.L. Correlation of foveal avascular zone size with foveal morphology in normal eyes using optical coherence tomography angiography. *Retina* **2015**, *35*, 2188–2195. [CrossRef]

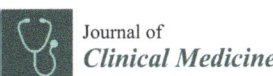

Review

Clinical Applications of Optical Coherence Tomography Angiography in Inherited Retinal Diseases: An Up-to-Date Review of the Literature

Claudio Iovino, Clemente Maria Iodice, Danila Pisani, Luciana Damiano, Valentina Di Iorio, Francesco Testa * and Francesca Simonelli

Eye Clinic, Multidisciplinary Department of Medical, Surgical and Dental Sciences, University of Campania Luigi Vanvitelli, 80131 Naples, Italy
* Correspondence: francesco.testa@unicampania.it

Abstract: Optical coherence tomography angiography (OCT-A) is a valuable imaging technique, allowing non-invasive, depth-resolved, motion-contrast, high-resolution images of both retinal and choroidal vascular networks. The imaging capabilities of OCT-A have enhanced our understanding of the retinal and choroidal alterations that occur in inherited retinal diseases (IRDs), a group of clinically and genetically heterogeneous disorders that may be complicated by several vascular conditions requiring a prompt diagnosis. In this review, we aimed to comprehensively summarize all clinical applications of OCT-A in the diagnosis and management of IRDs, highlighting significant vascular findings on retinitis pigmentosa, Stargardt disease, choroideremia, Best disease and other less common forms of retinal dystrophies. All advantages and limitations of this novel imaging modality will be also discussed.

Keywords: Best disease; choroideremia; inherited retinal diseases; optical coherence tomography angiography; retinitis pigmentosa; Stargardt disease

1. Introduction

Optical coherence tomography angiography (OCT-A) is a novel imaging technique that relies on the intrinsic movement of red blood cells (RBCs), allowing non-invasive, motion-contrast, high-resolution images of both retinal and choroidal vascular networks [1].

The retina is supplied by up to 4 layers of vessels: (1) the radial peripapillary capillary network, within the nerve fiber layer and located around the optic nerve head; (2) the superficial vascular plexus, within the ganglion cells layer; (3) the deep capillary complex, which comprises 2 capillary beds on both sides of the inner nuclear layer [2].

The choroid, conversely, consists of 3 layers of vessels: (1) the Haller layer, the outer, large-caliber layer of vessels; (2) the Sattler layer, the middle, smaller-diameter layer of vessels; (3) the choriocapillaris, which is the innermost and smallest layer of vessels [2].

OCT-A is able to clearly display several vascular alterations, including, among others, areas of macular telangiectasia, impaired perfusion, microaneurysms, capillary remodeling and neovascularization [3]. In contrast with conventional imaging modalities, the dye-free image acquisition of this method avoids the onset of typical side effects of fluorescein and indocyanine green angiography (FA and ICGA) [4,5].

More importantly, OCT-A allows depth-resolved analysis of retinal tissue that has never been available before [3]. OCT-A has been adopted to investigate a broad spectrum of retinal vascular diseases, ranging from diabetic retinopathy and retinal venous occlusion, up to age-related macular degeneration, and inflammatory and ocular oncology disorders [3]. Over the past 15 years, the retinal and choroidal imaging capabilities of OCT-A have been applied to further characterize primary and secondary alterations in inherited retinal diseases (IRDs). In this review of the literature, we aim to analyze and summarize all

Citation: Iovino, C.; Iodice, C.M.; Pisani, D.; Damiano, L.; Di Iorio, V.; Testa, F.; Simonelli, F. Clinical Applications of Optical Coherence Tomography Angiography in Inherited Retinal Diseases: An Up-to-Date Review of the Literature. *J. Clin. Med.* **2023**, *12*, 3170. https://doi.org/10.3390/jcm12093170

Academic Editor: Masayuki Akimoto

Received: 21 March 2023
Revised: 14 April 2023
Accepted: 26 April 2023
Published: 28 April 2023

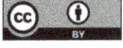

Copyright: © 2023 by the authors. Licensee MDPI, Basel, Switzerland. This article is an open access article distributed under the terms and conditions of the Creative Commons Attribution (CC BY) license (https://creativecommons.org/licenses/by/4.0/).

clinical applications of OCT-A in the diagnosis and management of IRDs and to discuss advantages and limitations of this imaging technique.

2. Optical Coherence Tomography Angiography Technical Aspects

OCT-A is an optical coherence tomography (OCT)-based imaging technique that enables the visualization of blood vessels within the eye, and it is built on the principle of OCT signal variation generated by the moving RBCs within the vessels [6–8]. Multiple scans are performed at the same location and the subsequent temporal changes of the OCT signal caused by the constant motion of the RBCs generate angiographic contrast, allowing visualization of the microvasculature [3].

Barton et al., in 2005, laid the foundation for this relatively new technology, which has only been commercially available since 2016 [9]. The authors adjusted analysis of speckles to produce an amplitude-based angiogram [9]. The speckle pattern stays relatively constant over time for static objects, while it changes for moving scatterers (i.e., erythrocytes) [9]. In 2009, Wang et al. introduced optical microangiography (OMAG), an imaging technique in which spatial frequency analysis of time-varying spectral interferograms was used to distinguish the signals backscattered by particles in motion from those backscattered by static objects, creating a high-resolution angiogram image [10]. Subsequently, in 2012, Jia et al. developed a more refined signal processing algorithm, named split-spectrum amplitude-decorrelation angiography (SSADA), which enhanced the signal-to-noise ratio of flow detection while reducing the pulsatile bulk-motion noise [11].

OCT-A may be captured with spectral domain OCT (SD-OCT), which, in commercial devices, employs a wavelength of ~840 nm, or with swept-source OCT (SS-OCT), which uses a longer wavelength of ~1050 nm [12].

While OCT is considered a cross-sectional imaging modality, OCT-A images are mainly studied with en face visualization. Currently, all commercially available OCT-A platforms allow the segmentation of the volumetric scans at specific depths through the definition of "slabs" [12].

FA and ICGA have been considered, so far, the gold standard for the evaluation of retinal and choroidal vasculature in vivo. Nevertheless, although dye injection is generally safe, serious allergic reactions may occur and these techniques are therefore considered invasive [12]. Moreover, the use of dyes in pregnant or breastfeeding women appears to be controversial [13,14].

OCT-A provides a non-invasive and fast analysis of choroidal and retinal microvascular circulation without the need for any dye injection. Moreover, it has the additional advantage of depth-resolution with better visualization of the deeper vascular layers [12].

3. Clinical Applications

3.1. OCT-A in Retinitis Pigmentosa

Most of the literature about the findings of OCT-A in retinitis pigmentosa (RP) converged to a common demonstration of retinal and choroidal vascular impairment. A summary of the data collected is reported in Table 1.

The mean follow-up ranged between 2 months and 36 months [12–31]. Overall, significant reductions in both the superficial capillary plexus (SCP) and deep capillary plexus (DCP) were observed in all the affected patients of the evaluated cohorts over time [12–31]. In addition, all the studies that explored the involvement of choriocapillaris (CC) demonstrated its significant impairment in RP patients [12,15–17,21–23,25,30,31]. Several authors focused on the variation of the foveal avascular zone (FAZ) area in RP patients, two-thirds of which described an increased avascular area [12,15,19,20,26,31], while the remaining third demonstrated its significant reduction [16,17,29]. Nakajima et al. and Alnawaiseh et al. explored an interesting association between the reduction in optic nerve head (ONH) vessel density (VD) in RP patients and the deterioration of the visual field mean deviation (MD) [15,27]. The authors demonstrated that the VD in both the radial peripapillary capillary network and ONH layers was significantly lower in patients rather than controls, significantly correlating with the MD and the cup/disc area ratio [15,27]. Mastropasqua et al. investigated the mean microperimetry (MP) retinal sensitivity between RP patients and healthy subjects and explored possible correlations with retinal perfusion density [25]. The authors found a significant reduction in retinal sensitivity in RP patients, compared to healthy controls, at 4°, 8° and 20° [25]. A significant positive correlation was also observed in RP patients between the perfusion density of the central 1.5 mm retina in either DCP and CC and microperimetry at 4° and 8°, meaning that a reduction in the perfusion density would be associated with a retinal sensitivity decrease [25]. Toto et al. demonstrated instead that parafoveal SCP and DCP VD were significantly correlated with mfERG values, while parafoveal CC VD correlated directly with the P1R2 amplitude, highlighting that vessel impairment may affect macular function [33].

A representative case of RP patient examined with OCT-A is shown in Figure 1.

Table 1. Optical coherence tomography angiography features in patients with retinitis pigmentosa.

Authors	Study	F-UP	N. Eyes	SCP VD	DCP VD	CC VD	CH VD	ONH/RPL VD	FAZ Area
Alnawaiseh [15]	P	NA	20	Reduced	Reduced	Reduced	/	Reduced	Increased
Arrigo [16]	P	12 MO	68	Reduced	Reduced	/	/	/	/
Atas [17]	R	NA	26	Reduced	Reduced	/	/	/	/
Attaallah [18]	P	3 MO	24	Reduced	Reduced	Reduced	/	/	Increased
Deutsch [19]	R	24 MO	29	Reduced	Reduced	Reduced	Reduced	/	Reduced
Giansanti [20]	R	13 MO	52	Reduced	Reduced	Reduced	Reduced	/	Reduced
Hagag [21]	P	NA	44	Reduced	Reduced	/	/	/	/
Jauregui [22]	R	15 MO	28	Reduced	Reduced	/	/	/	Increased
Koyanagi [23]	R	24 MO	73	Both Reduced	Both Reduced	/	/	/	Increased
Liu [24]	R	36 MO	53	/	/	Reduced	Reduced	/	/
Mastropasqua [25]	P	6 MO	20	Both Reduced	Both Reduced	Both Reduced	/	/	/
Miyata [26]	P	2 MO	43	/	/	Reduced	/	/	/
Nakajima [27]	R	NA	38	/	Reduced	/	/	Reduced	/
Nassisi [28]	R	9 MO	28	Reduced	Reduced	Reduced	/	/	/
Parodi [29]	R	8 MO	32	Reduced	Reduced	/	/	/	Increased
Shen [30]	P	10 MO	34	Reduced	Reduced	/	/	/	/
Sugahara [31]	R	NA	68	Reduced	Reduced	/	/	/	/
Takagi [32]	R	6 MO	50	Reduced	Reduced	/	/	/	Reduced
Toto [33]	R	NA	28	Reduced	Reduced	Reduced	/	/	/
Wang [34]	P	NA	40	Both Reduced	Both Reduced	Both Reduced			Increased

CC: choriocapillaris; CVI: choroidal vascularity index; CH: choroid; DCP: deep capillary plexus; F-UP: follow-up; FAZ: foveal avascular zone; MO: months; NA: not applicable; N.: number of; ONH: optic nerve head; P: prospective; R: retrospective; RPL: radial peripapillary layer; SCP: superficial capillary plexus; VD: vessel density. Results were significant for $p < 0.05$.

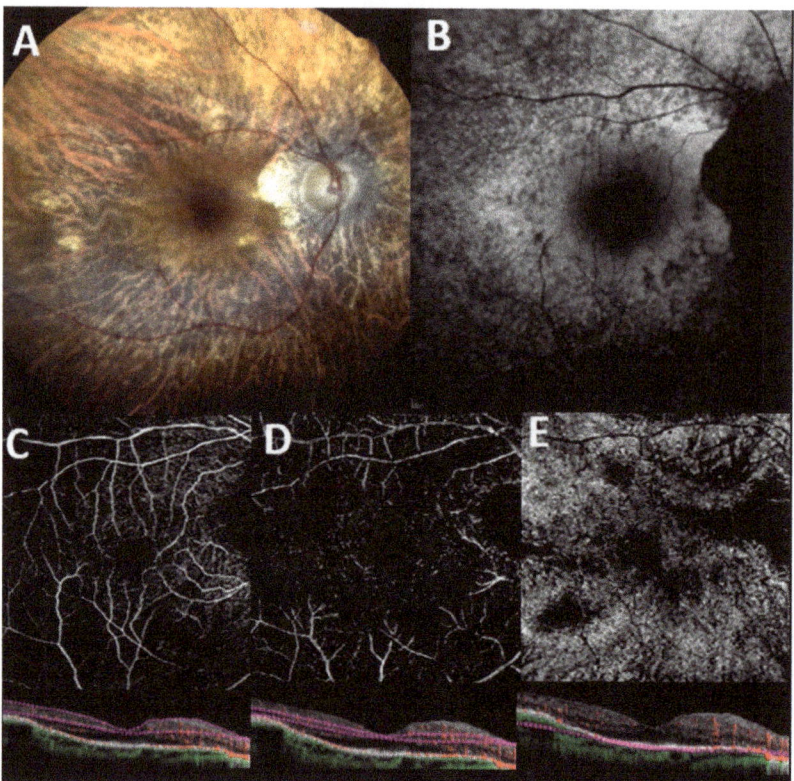

Figure 1. Multimodal imaging features in a patient with genetically confirmed retinitis pigmentosa. (**A**) Color fundus image displays pallor of the optic disc, attenuation of retinal vessels, extensive retinal atrophy, and pigmentary clumping in mid-periphery. (**B**) Blue-light autofluorescence (BAF) shows a granular hypoautofluorescence extending from the perifoveal region to the midperiphery. En face 6 × 6 optical coherence tomography angiography with corresponding B scan angio flow of superficial capillary plexus (**C**), deep capillary plexus (**D**), and choriocapillaris (**E**) with automatic segmentation. Flow voids areas are denoted in all retinal plexuses, and especially in the choriocapillaris, possibly related to either segmentation artifacts, outer retinal atrophy, or extremely reduced blood flow which fails to produce a signal (see corresponding B scans angio flow).

3.2. OCT-A in Choroideremia

Following animal model-based studies confirming the primary degeneration of RPE, photoreceptors and CC in choroideremia (CHM), Jain et al. showed, in a 6-month prospective study, that regional changes in CC density correlate with photoreceptor structural alterations in CHM [35–37]. They stratified their cohort in 3 groups based on the diagnosis of CHM, CHM carrier state, and healthy controls, demonstrating a significant difference of mean (±SD) CC density among them (82.9% ± 13.4%; 93.0% ± 3.8%; 98.2% ± 1.3%, respectively) [37]. Interestingly, the mean (±SD) CC density in affected eyes was also higher in regions with a preserved, rather than absent, ellipsoid zone (92.6% ± 5.8% vs. 75.9% ± 12.6%, mean difference, 16.7%; 95% CI, 12.1% to 21.3%; $p < 0.001$) [37]. En face outer retinal imaging in these eyes revealed an interesting degeneration pattern with a relatively unaffected central island of photoreceptors showing pseudopodial-like protrusions of surviving tissue, representing scrolled outer retina and outer retinal tubulations (ORTs) at the degeneration margins [38]. The formation of these features suggested that the underlying CC/Retinal pigment epithelium (RPE) would not adequately support the overlying retina, and that photoreceptor death could be a secondary process [37,38].

Abbouda et al. prospectively enrolled 26 eyes, 17 of which had a CHM diagnosis and 9 with a carrier status, focusing on superficial retinal vessel network (SRVN) and CC changes [39]. Both vascular networks appeared significantly reduced in CHM patients if compared to carriers and controls (SRVN: 12.93 ± 2.06 mm^2, 15.36 ± 0.60 mm^2, and 15.30 ± 1.35 mm^2, respectively; CC: 6.97 ± 5.26 mm^2, 21.65 ± 0.17 mm^2, and 21.36 ± 0.76 mm^2, respectively) [39]. Since the presence of a functional CC flow area was positively correlated to the SVRN, the authors postulated that a reduction in CC flow caused a compensatory reduction in SVRN circulation to keep retinal and choroidal circulations balanced [39]. In this regard, again, the missing step between the reduction in CC and SVRN flow could be the expression of reduced metabolic demand of that area of retina, due to the death of either RPE or photoreceptors [37,38].

Battaglia Parodi et al. prospectively examined a consecutive series of 12 eyes of 6 patients with a CHM diagnosis, and compared them with a group of healthy, age-matched controls with no ocular nor systemic disease [40]. The authors found no differences in SCP between cases and controls, both in terms of morphology and vessel density quantification, even by analyzing the preserved central island and external affected area separately [40]. Conversely, a statistically significant impairment was found with regard to DCP and CC. CHM patients displayed a reduced DCP vascular density in both the external macular area (0.017 ± 0.02; $p < 0.01$) and central preserved island (0.037 ± 0.02; $p < 0.01$) compared to controls (0.43 ± 0.03 and 0.43 ± 0.03, respectively) [40]. With regard to CC vessel densities, the peripheral macular area exhibited a significant reduction in patients (0.0 ± 0.0; $p < 0.01$) versus controls (0.49 ± 0.02) while no significant differences were demonstrated in the central preserved island [40]. This finding highlights the coexistence of two CC vessel density patterns, disclosing no changes in correspondence with preserved RPE islands, and an almost undetectable CC vessel density in external regions of substantial RPE deficiency. This supports the current belief that CC loss would occur secondary to RPE loss, not independently [40].

Murro et al. consecutively enrolled 14 eyes of 7 patients with CHM and 14 eyes of 7 healthy controls, demonstrating patients' significantly smaller FAZ in SCP and DCP ($19,899 \pm 8368$ and $24,398 \pm 86,11$, respectively) when compared to controls ($288,708 \pm 4505$ and $32,016 \pm 4821$, respectively) [41]. Quantitative analysis also disclosed statistically significant decreased SCP, DCP, and CC vascular densities, comparing patients with the age-matched control groups [41]. The same authors also explored OCT-A features of 6 CHM carriers (12 eyes), comparing their findings with 8 age-matched controls (16 eyes) [42]. The quantitative analysis of the inner retinal vasculature disclosed no significant differences in both SCP and DCP vessel densities compared to the control group [42]. Only CC showed a mild reduction in the vascular flow in the carrier versus control group (78.896 ± 13.972 vs. 80.008 ± 10.862; $p = 0.045$) [42]. Of note, OCT allowed the identification of the impaired RPE layer in the presence of a preserved central inner retinal and CC vascularization, suggesting that vascular impairment would follow RPE loss in the natural history of the disease [42].

Arrigo et al. designed an observational, cross-sectional clinical series with 7 CHM patients (14 eyes) and 7 age-matched controls (14 eyes), correlating retinal layer thickness with OCT-A findings [43]. Patients displayed significant differences with respect to DCP and CC vascular densities (F = 3941.3 and 655.9, respectively) [43]. Authors also stratified the cohort, assessing the vascular network densities independently based on chorioretinal atrophy areas and anatomically preserved islets [43]. They found that CHM patients displayed significantly lower DCP vascular density in both the atrophic and healthy areas when compared to healthy controls [43]. On the other hand, CC vascular density appeared to be impaired only in the atrophic region ($p < 0.001$) and not in the apparently preserved islet ($p = 0.19$), while SCP was found to be unaffected in both regions ($p > 0.05$) [43]. Interestingly, significant correlations were found between the reduction in DCP vascular density and the thinning of outer plexiform layer, inner nuclear layer, and inner plexiform layer [43].

The utility of OCT-A in the management of choroidal neovascularization (CNV) as a later-stage complication of CHM was also investigated [44,45]. The authors described evidence of a high-flow CC neovascular network in the context of a neighboring vascular attenuation, which regressed to a small juxtafoveal subretinal hyper-reflective lesion after prompt anti-VEGF treatment [44,45].

A representative case of a patient with CHM examined with OCT-A is shown in Figure 2.

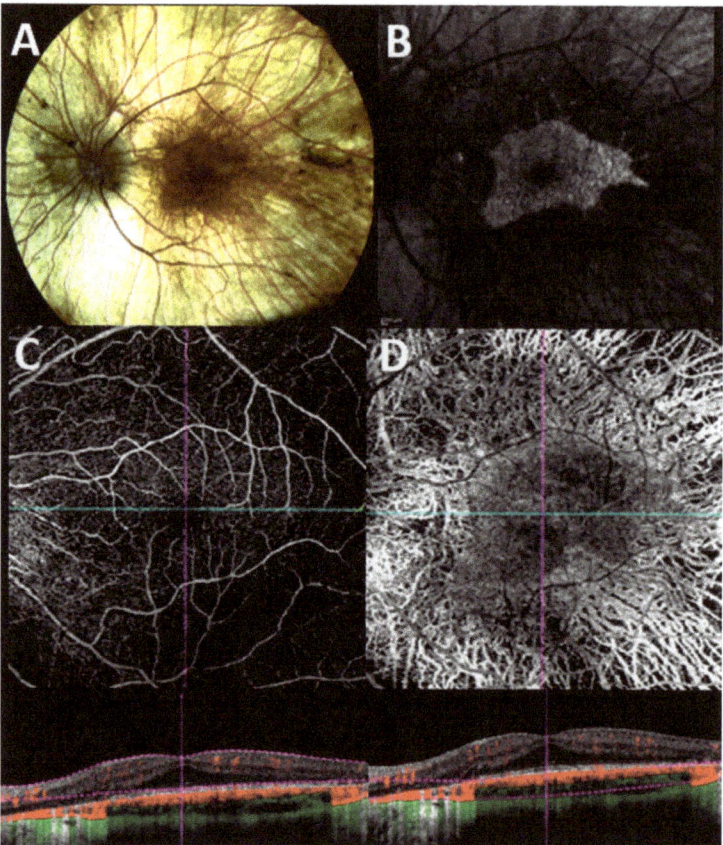

Figure 2. Multimodal imaging evaluation in a patient with genetically confirmed choroideremia. (**A**) Color fundus photograph shows extensive retinal degeneration with chorioretinal atrophy. (**B**) Blue light fundus autofluorescence shows typical patterns of a sharply demarcated macular area of remaining tissue (hyper/iso-autofluorescent) against surrounding atrophic RPE (hypoautofluorescent background). (**C**) En face 6 × 6 optical coherence tomography angiography (OCT-A) with corresponding B scan angio flow of the superficial capillary plexus (SCP) shows a preserved macular flow with some areas of flow reduction along the vascular arcade due to the underlying outer retinal atrophy. (**D**) En face 6 × 6 OCT-A with corresponding B scan angio flow of the choroidal slab shows a diffuse loss of vasculature with a relatively preserved island of flow in the foveal region.

3.3. OCT-A in Best Disease

Best vitelliform macular dystrophy (BVMD), also known as Best disease, is an autosomal-dominant inherited disorder caused by mutations in *BEST1* gene [46].

Vascular impairment in Best disease is described in the literature as a later-stage finding in the vitelliform and pseudohypopion stages; the subretinal deposits often cover the CC, showing an OCT-A dark area and, as the deposits disappear and the atrophy progresses, the CC would appear accordingly brighter and more granular [47]. This phase would coincide with the onset of vascular alterations and morphological changes [47]. Likewise, the choroid will change in thickness depending on the stage of the disease, generally appearing thicker in early stages and tending to get thinner in later phases [48].

In the literature, a reduction in vascular flow density is described in SCP and DCP layers, along with a significant FAZ enlargement [49]. Nevertheless, Mirshahi et al. described the presence of a capillary plexus across the FAZ, which could be consequent to a rise in the concentration of angiogenetic factors [50].

Vascular impairment was not only found in retinal vascular layers, but also in the CC. In particular, the CC flow density has been shown to decrease as the disease progresses [48].

Rarely, in about 10% of cases, CNV may occur, leading to a significant loss of vision [51]. Parodi et al. hypothesized a distinct mechanism of neovascularization according to the disease stage [52]. In particular, the early stages (stages 2 and 3) of BVMD are more likely to present with exudative CNV, characterized by higher values of both vessel tortuosity (VT) and vessel dispersion (VDisp) upon OCT-A examination [52]. On the contrary, late stages mainly display non-exudative CNV, with lower perfusion, VT, and VDisp. This would suggest that exudative CNV is associated with a faster growing neovascular network, whereas the non-exudative CNV may develop more slowly [52]. This finding was also confirmed by another study, which revealed the presence of two subgroups of neovascularization, not only in BVMD but also in other retinal diseases, such as central serous chorioretinopathy and age-related macular degeneration. Authors also found that the non-exudative CNV, more stable than the exudative CNV, would seem to not require anti-VEGF injections, as they would promote atrophy progression [53].

A recent study described that CNV onset may vary based on the disease stage, ranging from nearly 30% of cases in early phases and up to almost all cases in the atrophic stage [52].

3.4. OCT-A in Stargardt Disease

Stargardt disease (STGD1) is one of the most frequent macular dystrophies in young adults, commonly caused by mutations in the *ABCA4* gene [54]. Its prevalence is about 1:8000–10,000 [54].

STGD1 is characterized by the loss of photoreceptors and CC, with or without the presence of yellowish lipofuscin flecks extending beyond the vascular arcades to the medium and extreme retinal periphery [55].

The clinical phenotype of STGD1 has been shown to be heterogeneous. Indeed, OCT-A was used to classify the disease phenotypes representing the disease progression, based on different choroidal patterns: pattern (1) normal choroidal thickness, few localized foveal and perifoveal yellowish–whitish flecks; pattern (2) reduced Sattler or Haller layer, numerous yellow–white fundus lesions throughout the posterior pole; pattern (3) reduced Sattler and Haller layers + extensive atrophy area; pattern (4) pattern 3 features + choroidal caverns [56].

Mastropasqua and co-authors reported, in a prospective study, the OCT-A features of 24 eyes of 12 consecutive STGD1 patients in comparison with a healthy control group [57]. A quantitative analysis was carried out, revealing a diffused vascular attenuation, especially within the foveal and parafoveal SCP and DCP, in all patients of the STGD1 group [57]. In addition, the perifoveal anastomotic arcade was interrupted in all cases to varying extents. In 15 out of 20 eyes (75%), the CC displayed the presence of well-delineated black dots, probably as an epiphenomenon of non-perfused areas [57]. The parafoveal VD of SCP was significantly lower in the STGD1 group compared to the control group (46.34 ± 4.04 vs.

52.55 ± 2.94). Foveal and parafoveal VD of the DCP were significantly lower in the STGD1 group compared to the controls (37.52 ± 9.51 vs. 29.68 ± 7.42 and 47.38 ± 4.25 vs. 59.09 ± 2.79, respectively) [57]. The same applies for foveal and parafoveal CC, both significantly lower in the STGD1 group compared to healthy eyes (54.87 ± 24.84 vs. 27.51 ± 5.37 and 60.63 ± 6.46 vs. 67.11 ± 1.40, respectively) [57].

Della Volpe et al. focused their attention on evaluating, retrospectively, the metabolic function of 107 eyes of 56 STGD1 patients, assessed with retinal oximetry, and the relation with retinal microvascular changes [58]. The authors indeed demonstrated a significant enlargement of superficial FAZ and reduced mean arterial and venular oxygen saturations in their cohort [58].

Advanced stages of STGD1 often result in macular atrophy, frequently reported as misdiagnosed in the literature [59]. An interesting study operated a comparison between the OCT-A analysis of macular atrophy in patients with atrophic STGD1 and late-stage atrophic AMD [60]. The authors reported an extensive loss of CC in the central area with persisting tissue at its margins in STGD1 patients, whereas eyes with atrophic AMD displayed an area of RPE loss with still persistent, yet rarefied CC. This finding would suggest that CC breakdown might precede outer retinal degeneration in AMD, whereas RPE and outer retinal degeneration would precede and affect CC degeneration in STGD1 [60].

3.5. OCT-A in Miscellaneous Diseases

3.5.1. OCT-A in Gyrate Atrophy

Gyrate atrophy (GA) is an autosomal recessive chorioretinal degeneration caused by a mutation in the ornithine-δ-amino transferase (*OAT*) gene which produces a B6 enzyme that converts ornithine to glutamate [61]. GA is generally characterized by peripheral, circumferential, sharply demarcated, round patches of chorioretinal atrophy, and commonly associated with subcapsular cataract, cystoid macular edema, foveoschisis, and myopia [61]. OCT-A has been used to analyze microvascular abnormalities in patients with gyrate atrophy and cystoid macular edema. Authors reported a central dark-grey area without any evident vascular alteration attributed to a decreased signal due to the shadowing effect [62].

3.5.2. OCT-A in Bietti Dystrophy

Bietti dystrophy is an autosomic recessive chorioretinal degeneration characterized by *CYP4V2* mutations, featuring yellow–white retinal and corneal crystals and progressive degeneration and atrophy of the RPE [63]. OCT-A was described as an effective tool to allow a thorough evaluation of the choroid in patients affected, as reported by Myjata et al. [63]. Indeed, authors have prospectively demonstrated CC blood flow deficit in 12 out of 13 eyes included (92%) [63]. In addition, a significant decrease in DCP and SCP in patients with Bietti disease was reported as well. [64].

3.5.3. OCT-A in Leber Hereditary Optic Neuropathy

Leber hereditary optic neuropathy (LHON) is a mitochondrial inherited disorder, generally limited to the inner retina layers with characteristic loss of ganglion cells and their axons, parapapillary telangiectasia, and vascular focal tortuosity [65–67]. In the subacute stage of the disease, a characteristic reduction is reported in the radial peripapillary capillary density of both SCP and DCP, primarily localized in temporal sector, which corresponds to the papillomacular bundle [68–70]. Balducci et al., in a prospective observational study, first reported that the abovementioned microvascular changes in the temporal sector evaluated with OCT-A would be simultaneous to the GC-IPL thinning and would precede the retinal nerve fiber layer (RNFL) impairment assessed with OCT [69]. An association between the SCP and DCP vascular impairment and the RNFL reduction has also been investigated in several other published papers, which confirmed a significant association between these features, even more marked in late chronic stages [69–71].

3.5.4. OCT-A in X-Linked Retinoschisis

X-linked juvenile retinoschisis (XLRS) is a macular degenerative disease that occurs exclusively in males and is associated with mutations in the *RS1* gene [72]. Most studies report that the schisis is mainly localized at the inner nuclear layer (INL), followed by the outer plexiform layer (OPL), the outer nuclear layer (ONL), and the ganglion cell layer (CGL) in a smaller number of cases [73]. Several studies in the literature have examined the vascular structure by the means of OCT-A, reporting a substantial enlargement and thinning of the FAZ area, telangiectasias, and vascular abnormalities at the level of both SCP and DCP, the latter of which was associated with a BCVA reduction [73–76]. Han et al. hypothesize that vascular alterations could have a primary role in the pathogenesis or may be the result of an artifact due to structural change [74].

4. Limitations

Imaging the retinal and choroidal layers by means of OCT-A may be challenging due to several artifacts which may confound their evaluation. Among the various source of artifacts associated with OCT-A imaging, the three that most dramatically and significantly impact the flow analysis, especially of the CC layer, include: segmentation errors, projection artifacts, and shadowing artifacts [12].

This is particularly evident in patients with IRDs due to atrophy of the outer retinal layers and RPE and to the presence of CME. The CC presents a significant segmentation challenge as it is extremely thin, and segmentation errors can cause regions of CC to be displaced outside the boundaries of the en face slab [77].

Moreover, more significant retinal vessel projection artifacts may occur in the CC in disorders with RPE disruption/atrophy.

5. Conclusions

OCT-A has progressively been recognized as a useful modality to evaluate retinal and choroidal blood flow in patients with IRDs. A growing body of evidence highlights its effectiveness in both diagnosis and management of these patients. Nevertheless, the role of OCT-A in the clinical management of patients with IRDs is yet to be precisely determined. Further randomized prospective studies with longer follow-ups and larger sample sizes are warranted, as they may reveal further insights into the pathogenesis and natural history of such diseases.

6. Methods of Literature Search

We carried out a review of literature regarding the applications of OCT-A in inherited retinal diseases using PubMed and Embase databases to November 2022 with the following terms: OCT-A in inherited retinal diseases, OCT-A in retinitis pigmentosa, OCT-A in choroideremia, OCT-A in Best disease, OCT-A in Stargardt disease, OCT-A in gyrate atrophy, OCT-A in Bietti Dystrophy, OCT-A in Leber Hereditary Optic Neuropathy, OCT-A in X-linked Retinoschisis, and combination of these. All relevant publications written in English were sourced, including prospective and retrospective clinical studies, and laboratory experimental studies. We included case reports only if they contributed new and relevant information about applications of OCT-A in inherited retinal diseases.

Author Contributions: Conceptualization: C.I.; Methodology: C.M.I., L.D., D.P. and V.D.I.; Writing—original draft preparation: C.I., L.D. and D.P.; Writing—review and editing: C.I., C.M.I., F.T. and F.S.; Resources: C.I. and F.S.; Supervision: C.I., F.T. and F.S. All authors have read and agreed to the published version of the manuscript.

Funding: This research received no external funding.

Institutional Review Board Statement: Not applicable.

Informed Consent Statement: Not applicable.

Data Availability Statement: Data sharing is not applicable to this article as no datasets were generated or analyzed in the current article.

Conflicts of Interest: The authors declare no conflict of interest.

References

1. Spaide, R.F.; Fujimoto, J.G.; Waheed, N.K.; Sadda, S.R.; Staurenghi, G. Optical Coherence Tomography Angiography. *Prog. Retin. Eye Res.* **2018**, *64*, 1–55. [CrossRef] [PubMed]
2. Kim, S.J. Retina and Vitreous; American Academy of Ophthalmology: San Francisco, CA, USA, 2017.
3. Kashani, A.H.; Chen, C.-L.; Gahm, J.K.; Richter, G.M.; Rosenfeld, P.J.; Shi, Y.; Wang, R.K. Optical Coherence Tomography Angiography: A Comprehensive Review of Current Methods and Clinical Applications HHS Public Access. *Prog. Retin. Eye Res.* **2017**, *60*, 66–100. [CrossRef] [PubMed]
4. Novotny, H.R.; Alvis, D.L. A Method of Photographing Fluorescence in Circulating Blood in the Human Retina. *Circulation* **1961**, *24*, 82–86. [CrossRef] [PubMed]
5. Invernizzi, A.; Pellegrini, M.; Cornish, E.; Teo, K.Y.C.; Cereda, M.; Chabblani, J. Imaging the Choroid: From Indocyanine Green Angiography to Optical Coherence Tomography Angiography. *Asia-Pac. J. Ophthalmol.* **2020**, *9*, 335–348. [CrossRef]
6. Chen, C.-L.; Wang, R.K. Optical Coherence Tomography Based Angiography [Invited]. *Biomed. Opt. Express* **2017**, *8*, 1056. [CrossRef]
7. Zhang, A.; Zhang, Q.; Chen, C.-L.; Wang, R.K. Methods and Algorithms for Optical Coherence Tomography-Based Angiography: A Review and Comparison. *J. Biomed. Opt.* **2015**, *20*, 100901. [CrossRef]
8. Wang, R.K.; Jacques, S.L.; Ma, Z.; Hurst, S.; Hanson, S.R.; Gruber, A. Three Dimensional Optical Angiography. *Opt. Express* **2007**, *15*, 4083. [CrossRef]
9. Barton, J.K.; Stromski, S. Flow Measurement without Phase Information in Optical Coherence Tomography Images. *Opt. Express* **2005**, *13*, 5234. [CrossRef]
10. Wang, R.K.; An, L. Doppler Optical Micro-Angiography for Volumetric Imaging of Vascular Perfusion in Vivo. *Opt. Express* **2009**, *17*, 8926. [CrossRef]
11. Jia, Y.; Tan, O.; Tokayer, J.; Potsaid, B.; Wang, Y.; Liu, J.J.; Kraus, M.F.; Subhash, H.; Fujimoto, J.G.; Hornegger, J.; et al. Split-Spectrum Amplitude-Decorrelation Angiography with Optical Coherence Tomography. *Opt. Express* **2012**, *20*, 4710. [CrossRef]
12. Borrelli, E.; Sarraf, D.; Freund, K.B.; Sadda, S.R. OCT Angiography and Evaluation of the Choroid and Choroidal Vascular Disorders. *Prog. Retin. Eye Res.* **2018**, *67*, 30–55. [CrossRef] [PubMed]
13. Fineman, M.S.; Maguire, J.I.; Fineman, S.W.; Benson, W.E. Safety of Indocyanine Green Angiography during Pregnancy: A Survey of the Retina, Macula, and Vitreous Societies. *Arch. Ophthalmol.* **2001**, *119*, 353–355. [CrossRef] [PubMed]
14. Halperin, L.S.; Olk, R.J.; Soubrane, G.; Coscas, G. Safety of Fluorescein Angiography during Pregnancy. *Am. J. Ophthalmol.* **1990**, *109*, 563–566. [CrossRef] [PubMed]
15. Alnawaiseh, M.; Schubert, F.; Heiduschka, P.; Eter, N. Optical Coherence Tomography Angiography in Patients with Retinitis Pigmentosa. *Retina* **2019**, *39*, 210–217. [CrossRef] [PubMed]
16. Arrigo, A.; Aragona, E.; Perra, C.; Bianco, L.; Antropoli, A.; Saladino, A.; Berni, A.; Basile, G.; Pina, A.; Bandello, F.; et al. Characterizing Macular Edema in Retinitis Pigmentosa through a Combined Structural and Microvascular Optical Coherence Tomography Investigation. *Sci. Rep.* **2023**, *13*, 800. [CrossRef]
17. Ataş, F.; Kayabaşı, M.; Saatci, A.O. Vessel Density and Choroidal Vascularity Index in Patients with Bietti Crystalline Dystrophy and Retinitis Pigmentosa. *Photodiagnosis Photodyn. Ther.* **2022**, *40*, 103181. [CrossRef]
18. Attaallah, H.R.; Mohamed, A.A.M.; Hamid, M.A. Quantification of Macular Microvascular Changes in Retinitis Pigmentosa Using Optical Coherence Tomography Angiography. *Clin. Ophthalmol.* **2020**, *14*, 1705–1713. [CrossRef]
19. Deutsch, S.; Lommatzsch, A.; Weinitz, S.; Farmand, G.; Kellner, U. Optical Coherence Tomography Angiography (OCT-A) in Retinitis Pigmentosa and Macular Dystrophy Patients: A Retrospective Study. *Graefe's Arch. Clin. Exp. Ophthalmol.* **2022**, *260*, 1923–1931. [CrossRef]
20. Giansanti, F.; Vicini, G.; Sodi, A.; Nicolosi, C.; Bellari, L.; Virgili, G.; Rizzo, S.; Bacherini, D. Optical Coherence Tomography Angiography for the Evaluation of Retinal and Choroidal Vasculature in Retinitis Pigmentosa: A Monocentric Experience. *Diagnostics* **2022**, *12*, 1020. [CrossRef]
21. Hagag, A.M.; Wang, J.; Lu, K.; Harman, G.; Weleber, R.G.; Huang, D.; Yang, P.; Pennesi, M.E.; Jia, Y. Projection-Resolved Optical Coherence Tomographic Angiography of Retinal Plexuses in Retinitis Pigmentosa. *Am. J. Ophthalmol.* **2019**, *204*, 70–79. [CrossRef]
22. Jauregui, R.; Park, K.S.; Duong, J.K.; Mahajan, V.B.; Tsang, S.H. Quantitative Progression of Retinitis Pigmentosa by Optical Coherence Tomography Angiography. *Sci. Rep.* **2018**, *8*, 13130. [CrossRef] [PubMed]
23. Koyanagi, Y.; Murakami, Y.; Funatsu, J.; Akiyama, M.; Nakatake, S.; Fujiwara, K.; Tachibana, T.; Nakao, S.; Hisatomi, T.; Yoshida, S.; et al. Optical Coherence Tomography Angiography of the Macular Microvasculature Changes in Retinitis Pigmentosa. *Acta Ophthalmol.* **2018**, *96*, e59–e67. [CrossRef] [PubMed]
24. Liu, R.; Lu, J.; Liu, Q.; Wang, Y.; Cao, D.; Wang, J.; Wang, X.; Pan, J.; Ma, L.; Jin, C.; et al. Effect of Choroidal Vessel Density on the Ellipsoid Zone and Visual Function in Retinitis Pigmentosa Using Optical Coherence Tomography Angiography. *Investig. Ophthalmol. Vis. Sci.* **2019**, *60*, 4328–4335. [CrossRef] [PubMed]

25. Mastropasqua, R.; D'Aloisio, R.; de Nicola, C.; Ferro, G.; Senatore, A.; Libertini, D.; di Marzio, G.; di Nicola, M.; di Martino, G.; di Antonio, L.; et al. Widefield Swept Source OCTA in Retinitis Pigmentosa. *Diagnostics* **2020**, *10*, 50. [CrossRef] [PubMed]
26. Miyata, M.; Oishi, A.; Hasegawa, T.; Oishi, M.; Numa, S.; Otsuka, Y.; Uji, A.; Kadomoto, S.; Hata, M.; Ikeda, H.O.; et al. Concentric Choriocapillaris Flow Deficits in Retinitis Pigmentosa Detected Using Wide-Angle Swept-Source Optical Coherence Tomography Angiography. *Investig. Ophthalmol. Vis. Sci.* **2019**, *60*, 1044–1049. [CrossRef] [PubMed]
27. Nakajima, K.; Inoue, T.; Maruyama-Inoue, M.; Yanagi, Y.; Kadonosono, K.; Ogawa, A.; Hashimoto, Y.; Azuma, K.; Terao, R.; Asaoka, R.; et al. Relationship between the Vessel Density around the Optic Nerve Head and Visual Field Deterioration in Eyes with Retinitis Pigmentosa. *Graefes Arch. Clin. Exp. Ophthalmol.* **2022**, *260*, 1097–1103. [CrossRef]
28. Nassisi, M.; Lavia, C.; Mohand-Said, S.; Smirnov, V.; Antonio, A.; Condroyer, C.; Sancho, S.; Varin, J.; Gaudric, A.; Zeitz, C.; et al. Near-Infrared Fundus Autofluorescence Alterations Correlate with Swept-Source Optical Coherence Tomography Angiography Findings in Patients with Retinitis Pigmentosa. *Sci. Rep.* **2021**, *11*, 3180. [CrossRef]
29. Parodi, M.B.; Cicinelli, M.V.; Rabiolo, A.; Pierro, L.; Gagliardi, M.; Bolognesi, G.; Bandello, F. Vessel Density Analysis in Patients with Retinitis Pigmentosa by Means of Optical Coherence Tomography Angiography. *Br. J. Ophthalmol.* **2017**, *101*, 428–432. [CrossRef]
30. Shen, C.; Li, Y.; Wang, Q.; Chen, Y.N.; Li, W.; Wei, W. Choroidal Vascular Changes in Retinitis Pigmentosa Patients Detected by Optical Coherence Tomography Angiography. *BMC Ophthalmol.* **2020**, *20*, 384. [CrossRef]
31. Sugahara, M.; Miyata, M.; Ishihara, K.; Gotoh, N.; Morooka, S.; Ogino, K.; Hasegawa, T.; Hirashima, T.; Yoshikawa, M.; Hata, M.; et al. Optical Coherence Tomography Angiography to Estimate Retinal Blood Flow in Eyes with Retinitis Pigmentosa. *Sci. Rep.* **2017**, *7*, 46396. [CrossRef]
32. Takagi, S.; Hirami, Y.; Takahashi, M.; Fujihara, M.; Mandai, M.; Miyakoshi, C.; Tomita, G.; Kurimoto, Y. Optical Coherence Tomography Angiography in Patients with Retinitis Pigmentosa Who Have Normal Visual Acuity. *Acta Ophthalmol.* **2018**, *96*, e636–e642. [CrossRef] [PubMed]
33. Toto, L.; Borrelli, E.; Mastropasqua, R.; Senatore, A.; di Antonio, L.; di Nicola, M.; Carpineto, P.; Mastropasqua, L. Macular Features in Retinitis Pigmentosa: Correlations Among Ganglion Cell Complex Thickness, Capillary Density, and Macular Function. *Investig. Ophthalmol. Vis. Sci.* **2016**, *57*, 6360–6366. [CrossRef] [PubMed]
34. Wang, X.N.; Zhao, Q.; Li, D.J.; Wang, Z.Y.; Chen, W.; Li, Y.F.; Cui, R.; Shen, L.; Wang, R.K.; Peng, X.Y.; et al. Quantitative Evaluation of Primary Retinitis Pigmentosa Patients Using Colour Doppler Flow Imaging and Optical Coherence Tomography Angiography. *Acta Ophthalmol.* **2019**, *97*, e993–e997. [CrossRef] [PubMed]
35. Tolmachova, T.; Wavre-Shapton, S.T.; Barnard, A.R.; MacLaren, R.E.; Futter, C.E.; Seabra, M.C. Retinal Pigment Epithelium Defects Accelerate Photoreceptor Degeneration in Cell Type-Specific Knockout Mouse Models of Choroideremia. *Investig. Ophthalmol. Vis. Sci.* **2010**, *51*, 4913–4920. [CrossRef] [PubMed]
36. Tolmachova, T.; Anders, R.; Abrink, M.; Bugeon, L.; Dallman, M.J.; Futter, C.E.; Ramalho, J.S.; Tonagel, F.; Tanimoto, N.; Seeliger, M.W.; et al. Independent Degeneration of Photoreceptors and Retinal Pigment Epithelium in Conditional Knockout Mouse Models of Choroideremia. *J. Clin. Investig.* **2006**, *116*, 386–394. [CrossRef] [PubMed]
37. Jain, N.; Jia, Y.; Gao, S.S.; Zhang, X.; Weleber, R.G.; Huang, D.; Pennesi, M.E. Optical Coherence Tomography Angiography in Choroideremia: Correlating Choriocapillaris Loss with Overlying Degeneration. *JAMA Ophthalmol.* **2016**, *134*, 697–702. [CrossRef]
38. Schaal, K.B.; Freund, K.B.; Litts, K.M.; Zhang, Y.; Messinger, J.D.; Curcio, C.A. Outer Retinal Tubulation in Advanced Age-Related Macular Degeneration: Optical Coherence Tomographic Findings Correspond to Histology. *Retina* **2015**, *35*, 1339–1350. [CrossRef]
39. Abbouda, A.; Dubis, A.M.; Webster, A.R.; Moosajee, M. Identifying Characteristic Features of the Retinal and Choroidal Vasculature in Choroideremia Using Optical Coherence Tomography Angiography. *Eye* **2018**, *32*, 563–571. [CrossRef]
40. Battaglia Parodi, M.; Arrigo, A.; MacLaren, R.E.; Aragona, E.; Toto, L.; Mastropasqua, R.; Manitto, M.P.; Bandello, F. Vascular Alterations Revealed with Optical Coherence Tomography Angiography in Patients with Choroideremia. *Retina* **2019**, *39*, 1200–1205. [CrossRef]
41. Murro, V.; Mucciolo, D.P.; Giorgio, D.; Sodi, A.; Passerini, I.; Virgili, G.; Rizzo, S. Optical Coherence Tomography Angiography (OCT-A) in Young Choroideremia (CHM) Patients. *Ophthalmic Genet.* **2019**, *40*, 201–206. [CrossRef]
42. Murro, V.; Mucciolo, D.P.; Giorgio, D.; Sodi, A.; Passerini, I.; Virgili, G.; Rizzo, S. Optical Coherence Tomography Angiography (OCT-A) in Choroideremia (CHM) Carriers. *Ophthalmic Genet.* **2020**, *41*, 146–151. [CrossRef] [PubMed]
43. Arrigo, A.; Romano, F.; Parodi, M.B.; Charbel Issa, P.; Birtel, J.; Bandello, F.; MacLaren, R.E. Reduced Vessel Density in Deep Capillary Plexus Correlates with Retinal Layer Thickness in Choroideremia. *Br. J. Ophthalmol.* **2021**, *105*, 687–693. [CrossRef] [PubMed]
44. Patel, R.C.; Gao, S.S.; Zhang, M.; Alabduljalil, T.; Al-Qahtani, A.; Weleber, R.G.; Yang, P.; Jia, Y.; Huang, D.; Pennesi, M.E. Optical Coherence Tomography Angiography of Choroidal Neovascularization in Four Inherited Retinal Dystrophies. *Retina* **2016**, *36*, 2339–2347. [CrossRef]
45. Ranjan, R.; Verghese, S.; Salian, R.; Manayath, G.J.; Saravanan, V.R.; Narendran, V. OCT Angiography for the Diagnosis and Management of Choroidal Neovascularization Secondary to Choroideremia. *Am. J. Ophthalmol. Case Rep.* **2021**, *22*, 101042. [CrossRef]
46. Sodi, A.; Passerini, I.; Murro, V.; Caputo, R.; Bacci, G.M.; Bodoj, M.; Torricelli, F.; Menchini, U. BEST1 Sequence Variants in Italian Patients with Vitelliform Macular Dystrophy. *Mol. Vis.* **2012**, *18*, 2736–2748. [PubMed]

47. Jauregui, R.; Parmann, R.; Nuzbrokh, Y.; Tsang, S.H.; Sparrow, J.R. Stage-Dependent Choriocapillaris Impairment in Best Vitelliform Macular Dystrophy Characterized by Optical Coherence Tomography Angiography. *Sci. Rep.* **2021**, *11*, 14300. [CrossRef]
48. Wang, X.N.; You, Q.S.; Li, Q.; Li, Y.; Mao, Y.; Hu, F.; Zhao, H.Y.; Tsai, F.F.; Peng, X.Y. Findings of Optical Coherence Tomography Angiography in Best Vitelliform Macular Dystrophy. *Ophthalmic Res.* **2018**, *60*, 214–220. [CrossRef] [PubMed]
49. Battaglia Parodi, M.; Romano, F.; Cicinelli, M.V.; Rabiolo, A.; Arrigo, A.; Pierro, L.; Iacono, P.; Bandello, F. Retinal Vascular Impairment in Best Vitelliform Macular Dystrophy Assessed by Means of Optical Coherence Tomography Angiography. *Am. J. Ophthalmol.* **2018**, *187*, 61–70. [CrossRef] [PubMed]
50. Mirshahi, A.; Lashay, A.; Masoumi, A.; Abrishami, M. Optical Coherence Tomography Angiography in Best Vitelliform Macular Dystrophy. *J. Curr. Ophthalmol.* **2019**, *31*, 442–445. [CrossRef]
51. Da, S.; Maurizio, P.; Parodi, B.; Toto, L.; Ravalico, G. Occult Choroidal Neovascularization in Adult-Onset Foveomacular Vitelliform Dystrophy. *Ophthalmologica* **2001**, *215*, 412–414.
52. Parodi, M.B.; Arrigo, A.; Bandello, F. Optical Coherence Tomography Angiography Quantitative Assessment of Macular Neovascularization in Best Vitelliform Macular Dystrophy. *Investig. Ophthalmol. Vis. Sci.* **2020**, *61*, 61. [CrossRef]
53. Arrigo, A.; Bordato, A.; Aragona, E.; Amato, A.; Viganò, C.; Bandello, F.; Battaglia Parodi, M. Macular Neovascularization in AMD, CSC and Best Vitelliform Macular Dystrophy: Quantitative OCTA Detects Distinct Clinical Entities. *Eye* **2021**, *35*, 3266–3276. [CrossRef] [PubMed]
54. Tsang, S.H.; Sharma, T. Stargardt Disease. In *Advances in Experimental Medicine and Biology*; Springer: New York, NY, USA, 2018; Volume 1085, pp. 139–151.
55. Arrigo, A.; Romano, F.; Aragona, E.; di Nunzio, C.; Sperti, A.; Bandello, F.; Parodi, M.B. Octa-Based Identification of Different Vascular Patterns in Stargardt Disease. *Transl. Vis. Sci. Technol.* **2019**, *8*, 26. [CrossRef] [PubMed]
56. Arrigo, A.; Grazioli, A.; Romano, F.; Aragona, E.; Bordato, A.; di Nunzio, C.; Sperti, A.; Bandello, F.; Parodi, M.B. Choroidal Patterns in Stargardt Disease: Correlations with Visual Acuity and Disease Progression. *J. Clin. Med.* **2019**, *8*, 1388. [CrossRef] [PubMed]
57. Mastropasqua, R.; Toto, L.; Borrelli, E.; Di Antonio, L.; Mattei, P.A.; Senatore, A.; Di Nicola, M.; Mariotti, C. Optical Coherence Tomography Angiography Findings in Stargardt Disease. *PLoS ONE* **2017**, *12*, e0170343. [CrossRef] [PubMed]
58. Della Volpe Waizel, M.; Scholl, H.P.N.; Todorova, M.G. Microvascular and Metabolic Alterations in Retinitis Pigmentosa and Stargardt Disease. *Acta Ophthalmol.* **2021**, *99*, e1396–e1404. [CrossRef]
59. Birnbach, C.D.; Järveläinen, M.; Possin, D.E.; Milam, A.H. Histopathology and Immunocytochemistry of the Neurosensory Retina in Fundus Flavimaculatus. *Ophthalmology* **1994**, *101*, 1211–1219. [CrossRef]
60. Müller, P.L.; Pfau, M.; Möller, P.T.; Nadal, J.; Schmid, M.; Lindner, M.; de Sisternes, L.; Stöhr, H.; Weber, B.H.F.; Neuhaus, C.; et al. Choroidal Flow Signal in Late-Onset Stargardt Disease and Age-Related Macular Degeneration: An OCT-Angiography Study. *Investig. Ophthalmol. Vis. Sci.* **2018**, *59*, AMD122–AMD131. [CrossRef]
61. Mansour, A.M.; Elnahry, A.G.; Tripathy, K.; Foster, R.E.; Mehanna, C.J.; Vishal, R.; Çavdarlı, C.; Arrigo, A.; Parodi, M.B. Analysis of Optical Coherence Angiography in Cystoid Macular Oedema Associated with Gyrate Atrophy. *Eye* **2021**, *35*, 1766–1774. [CrossRef]
62. Zhioua Braham, I.; Ammous, I.; Maalej, R.; Boukari, M.; Mili Boussen, I.; Errais, K.; Zhioua, R. Multimodal Imaging of Foveoschisis and Macular Pseudohole Associated with Gyrate Atrophy: A Family Report. *BMC Ophthalmol.* **2018**, *18*, 89. [CrossRef]
63. Miyata, M.; Oishi, A.; Hasegawa, T.; Ishihara, K.; Oishi, M.; Ogino, K.; Sugahara, M.; Hirashima, T.; Hata, M.; Yoshikawa, M.; et al. Choriocapillaris Flow Deficit in Bietti Crystalline Dystrophy Detected Using Optical Coherence Tomography Angiography. *Br. J. Ophthalmol.* **2018**, *102*, 1208–1212. [CrossRef] [PubMed]
64. Tiryaki Demir, S.; Keles Yesiltas, S.; Kacar, H.; Akbas, E.B.; Guven, D. Optical Coherence Tomography and Optical Coherence Tomography Angiography Imaging in Bietti Crystalline Dystrophy. *Ophthalmic Genet.* **2020**, *41*, 194–197. [CrossRef] [PubMed]
65. Takayama, K.; Ito, Y.; Kaneko, H.; Kataoka, K.; Ra, E.; Terasaki, H. Optical Coherence Tomography Angiography in Leber Hereditary Optic Neuropathy. *Acta Ophthalmol.* **2017**, *95*, e344–e345. [CrossRef] [PubMed]
66. Ghasemi Falavarjani, K.; Tian, J.J.; Akil, H.; Garcia, G.A.; Sadda, S.R.; Sadun, A.A. Swept-Source Optical Coherence Tomography Angiography of the Optic Disk in Optic Neuropathy. *Retina* **2016**, *36*, S168–S177. [CrossRef]
67. Gaier, E.D.; Gittinger, J.W.; Cestari, D.M.; Miller, J.B. Peripapillary Capillary Dilation in Leber Hereditary Optic Neuropathy Revealed by Optical Coherence Tomographic Angiography. *JAMA Ophthalmol.* **2016**, *134*, 1332–1334. [CrossRef]
68. Borrelli, E.; Balasubramanian, S.; Triolo, G.; Barboni, P.; Sadda, S.V.R.; Sadun, A.A. Topographic Macular Microvascular Changes and Correlation With Visual Loss in Chronic Leber Hereditary Optic Neuropathy. *Am. J. Ophthalmol.* **2018**, *192*, 217–228. [CrossRef]
69. Balducci, N.; Cascavilla, M.L.; Ciardella, A.; la Morgia, C.; Triolo, G.; Parisi, V.; Bandello, F.; Sadun, A.A.; Carelli, V.; Barboni, P. Peripapillary Vessel Density Changes in Leber's Hereditary Optic Neuropathy: A New Biomarker. *Clin. Exp. Ophthalmol.* **2018**, *46*, 1055–1062. [CrossRef]
70. Yu, Y.; Xu, H.; Huang, Y.; Gu, R.; Zong, Y.; Zhu, H.; Wang, M. Changes in Retinal Perfusion in Leber's Hereditary Optic Neuropathy: An Optical Coherence Tomography-Angiography Study. *Ophthalmic Res.* **2021**, *64*, 863–870. [CrossRef]
71. Kousal, B.; Kolarova, H.; Meliska, M.; Bydzovsky, J.; Diblik, P.; Kulhanek, J.; Votruba, M.; Honzik, T.; Liskova, P. Peripapillary Microcirculation in Leber Hereditary Optic Neuropathy. *Acta Ophthalmol.* **2019**, *97*, e71–e76. [CrossRef]

72. Molday, R.S.; Kellner, U.; Weber, B.H.F. X-Linked Juvenile Retinoschisis: Clinical Diagnosis, Genetic Analysis, and Molecular Mechanisms. *Prog. Retin. Eye Res.* **2012**, *31*, 195–212. [CrossRef]
73. Padrón-Pérez, N.; Català-Mora, J.; Díaz, J.; Arias, L.; Prat, J.; Caminal, J.M. Swept-Source and Optical Coherence Tomography Angiography in Patients with X-Linked Retinoschisis. *Eye* **2018**, *32*, 707–715. [CrossRef] [PubMed]
74. Han, I.C.; Whitmore, S.S.; Critser, D.B.; Lee, S.Y.; DeLuca, A.P.; Daggett, H.T.; Affatigato, L.M.; Mullins, R.F.; Tucker, B.A.; Drack, A.V.; et al. Wide-Field Swept-Source OCT and Angiography in X-Linked Retinoschisis. *Ophthalmol. Retina* **2019**, *3*, 178–185. [CrossRef] [PubMed]
75. Stringa, F.; Tsamis, E.; Papayannis, A.; Chwiejczak, K.; Jalil, A.; Biswas, S.; Ahmad, H.; Stanga, P.E. Segmented Swept Source Optical Coherence Tomography Angiography Assessment of the Perifoveal Vasculature in Patients with X-Linked Juvenile Retinoschisis: A Serial Case Report. *Int. Med. Case Rep. J.* **2017**, *10*, 329–335. [CrossRef] [PubMed]
76. Romano, F.; Arrigo, A.; Ch'Ng, S.W.; Parodi, M.B.; Manitto, M.P.; Martina, E.; Bandello, F.; Stanga, P.E. Capillary Network Alterations in X-Linked Retinoschisis Imaged on Optical Coherence Tomography Angiography. *Retina* **2019**, *39*, 1761–1767. [CrossRef]
77. Ghasemi Falavarjani, K.; Al-Sheikh, M.; Akil, H.; Sadda, S.R. Image Artefacts in Swept-Source Optical Coherence Tomography Angiography. *Br. J. Ophthalmol.* **2017**, *101*, 564–568. [CrossRef]

Disclaimer/Publisher's Note: The statements, opinions and data contained in all publications are solely those of the individual author(s) and contributor(s) and not of MDPI and/or the editor(s). MDPI and/or the editor(s) disclaim responsibility for any injury to people or property resulting from any ideas, methods, instructions or products referred to in the content.

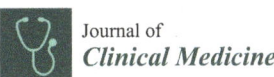

Review

Application of Deep Learning to Retinal-Image-Based Oculomics for Evaluation of Systemic Health: A Review

Jo-Hsuan Wu [1] and Tin Yan Alvin Liu [2,*]

[1] Shiley Eye Institute and Viterbi Family Department of Ophthalmology, University of California, San Diego, CA 92093, USA
[2] Wilmer Eye Institute, Johns Hopkins University, Baltimore, MD 21287, USA
* Correspondence: tliu25@jhmi.edu

Abstract: The retina is a window to the human body. Oculomics is the study of the correlations between ophthalmic biomarkers and systemic health or disease states. Deep learning (DL) is currently the cutting-edge machine learning technique for medical image analysis, and in recent years, DL techniques have been applied to analyze retinal images in oculomics studies. In this review, we summarized oculomics studies that used DL models to analyze retinal images—most of the published studies to date involved color fundus photographs, while others focused on optical coherence tomography images. These studies showed that some systemic variables, such as age, sex and cardiovascular disease events, could be consistently robustly predicted, while other variables, such as thyroid function and blood cell count, could not be. DL-based oculomics has demonstrated fascinating, "super-human" predictive capabilities in certain contexts, but it remains to be seen how these models will be incorporated into clinical care and whether management decisions influenced by these models will lead to improved clinical outcomes.

Keywords: oculomics; artificial intelligence; machine learning; deep learning; retinal imaging; color fundus photograph; optical coherence tomography; systemic diseases; cardiovascular diseases; neurodegenerative diseases

1. Introduction

The retina is considered a window to the human body [1–4], as many systemic conditions have ocular manifestations, especially in the retina. The extensive correlations between retinal findings and systemic conditions can be attributed to the facts that the human retina is a direct extension of the central nervous system during embryonic development [5], and the retina is one of the most vascularized and metabolically active organs in the human body [6]. Characterization and quantification of retinal-systemic correlations is particularly valuable for gaining new insights, especially since the retina can be conveniently and readily imaged non-invasively using a variety of technologies. The term "oculomics" is coined to describe the clinical insights provided by correlating ophthalmic biomarkers with systemic health and diseases [1,7].

The most common retinal imaging modalities used in oculomics are color fundus photography and optical coherence tomography (OCT). Briefly, OCT performs high-resolution cross-sectional imaging of tissue structures in situ and in real time by measuring the time delay of light echoed from the tissue under examination [8,9]. The most common groups of diseases studied in oculomics are cardiovascular diseases (CVD) and neurodegenerative diseases (NDD) [1,10,11].

Oculomics studies concerning CVD typically involve color fundus photographs. For example, prior studies have shown that retinal vascular morphologies, such as vessel caliber and tortuosity, can help predict CVD risk factors [12], CVD mortality [13,14], and various major CVD events [15–18]. Similarly, retinal microvascular changes have been

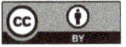

linked to higher risks of other systemic vascular diseases, such as kidney diseases and preeclampsia [19–21].

Oculomics studies concerning NDD typically involve OCTs. For example, retinal thickness measurements based on OCT have been used to diagnose and monitor multiple sclerosis (MS) [22–24]. Other studies have demonstrated an association between a thinner retinal nerve fiber layer (RNFL) and the diagnosis of Alzheimer's disease (AD) [25–29], which accounts for more than 60% of clinical dementia. A major area of OCT-based oculomics is the early detection of pre-clinical NDDs.

Historically, retinal image annotation and feature labeling were performed either manually by humans or semi-automatically in oculomics. The process is time-consuming, labor-intensive and limited by intra/inter-reader imprecision. Recently, the advent of deep learning (DL) has revolutionized the field of oculomics. Briefly, DL, a subtype of machine learning (ML), is a representation learning method that uses multilayered neural networks (NN) to reiteratively adjust parameters and enhance performance [30–33]. DL is superior to classical ML techniques in image analysis, and has emerged as the leading ML technique for medical image classification.

Medical subspecialities such as ophthalmology, with access to a large amount of imaging data, have been at the forefront of the DL revolution. Notably, DL has been shown to be on par with human experts in classifying various retinal diseases such as age-related macular degeneration and diabetic retinopathy [33–39], and the first FDA-approved fully autonomous system in any medical field is a DL-based system to detect diabetic retinopathy from color fundus photographs [40].

The retinal-systemic associations in oculomics were traditionally established using conventional statistical models or classical ML techniques. Given that oculomics primarily involves correlating ophthalmic biomarkers captured in retinal imaging with systemic conditions and that DL is the leading ML technique to analyze retinal images, the goal of this review is to summarize the latest literature in DL-based oculomics involving color fundus photography and OCT.

2. Literature Search Methods

The PubMed and Google Scholar databases were searched for published studies through July 2022, using individual and combinative search terms relevant to the this review. Major key words used included: (1) Deep learning-associated: "deep learning", "machine learning", and "neural network"; (2) Retinal imaging-associated: "ocular biomarkers", "oculomics", "ocular imaging", "retinal imaging", "fundus photographs", "optical coherence tomography"; (3) Systemic disease/health-associated: "age", "sex", "demographic", "systemic disease", "systemic biomarkers", "cardiovascular disease", "neurodegenerative disease", "stroke", "multiple sclerosis", "atherosclerosis", "blood pressure", "myocardial ischemia", "dementia", "Alzheimers disease", "diabetes", "renal disease", "kidney disease", etc.

No filter for publication year, language, or study type was applied. Reference of identified records were also checked. Studies applying DL on retinal-image-based oculomics to assess, predict, or diagnose systemic diseases and health biomarkers were considered relevant to the current review. Abstracts of non-English articles with relevant information were also included.

3. Results and Discussion

The following text is organized based on the imaging modality (fundus photography first, then OCT), and each sub-section is organized by the systemic parameter considered, with CVDs and their risk factors being the major focus.

3.1. Retinal Fundus Photography

Using retinal color fundus photographs from the UK Biobank and EyePACS, Poplin et al. published one of the first oculomics studies that demonstrated the ability of DL to predict systemic disease states and biomarkers [41]. In their study, a deep neural network

(NN) showed reasonably robust performance in predicting major CVD events with an area-under-the curve (AUC) of the operating characteristic curve of 0.70. For reference, an AUC of 1.0 indicates perfect predictions, while an AUC of 0.5 indicates predictions no better than random chance. The deep NN was also capable of robust prediction of age (mean absolute error [MAE] $\leq$ 3.3 years), sex (AUC = 0.97), and smoking status (AUC = 0.71), etc. Regions of the color fundus photographs most activated during decision making by the deep NN were highlighted using attention maps [41]. For example, strong activation centered on the retinal blood vessels was seen during prediction for age and smoking status, while strong activation at the optic disc, retinal blood vessels and macula was seen during prediction for gender.

3.1.1. Risk Assessment of CVD

Chang et al. presented a model that could generate a fundus atherosclerosis score (FAS) using DL-based retinal image analysis. The DL-generated FAS was then compared to the ground truth: a physician-graded score based on carotid ultrasonographic images. The DL model achieved an AUC of 0.71 in predicting the presence of carotid atherosclerosis [42]. Furthermore, by using the FAS to risk stratify patients, the authors found that cases in the top tertile (FAS > 0.66) had a significantly increased risk (hazard ratio = 8.33) of CVD mortality as compared to cases in the bottom tertile (FAS < 0.33). A similar CVD risk stratification study was performed by Son et al. [43]. They presented a model that could generate a coronary artery calcium score (CACS), by using DL-based retinal image analysis. The DL-generated CACS was compared to the cardiac computed tomography-derived CACS, and the model achieved an AUC > 0.82 in identifying cases with high CACS (CACS > 100).

Khan et al., the DL model was trained to predict the presence of cardiac diseases from fundus photographs. With the electronic health record (EHR) as the ground truth, their model reached an AUC of 0.7 [44]. In another study, Cheung et al. used convolutional neural network (CNN) to segment the retinal vessels from fundus photographs and measured the vessel calibers [45]. They correlated the vessel calibers generated from DL-based segmentation with incident CVD events (defined as newly diagnosed clinical stroke, myocardial infarction or CVD mortality in EHR), and found that narrower calibers at certain vascular zones were associated with increased incident CVD risk. Lastly, a recent Chinese study trained a DL model to predict 10-year ischemic CVD risk using retinal image analysis [46]. Their estimation was compared with the calculation by a previously validated 10-year Chinese CVD risk prediction model, and an AUC of 0.86 and 0.88 was reported for predicting 10-year ischemic CVD risk $\geq$5% and $\geq$7.5%, respectively.

3.1.2. Blood Pressure and Hypertension

In the study by Poplin et al., the DL model predicted diastolic BP (DBP) and systolic BP (SBP) with an MAE of 6.42 mmHg and 11.23 mmHg, respectively [41]. Subsequent studies published by different groups of authors showed similar results in that, in general, MAE of DBP (range: 6–9 mmHg) was smaller than that of SBP (range: 9–15 mmHg) [47,48]. Of note, a weak-to-moderate R^2 ranged from 0.20 to 0.50 was observed for most DL models for BP prediction. Other studies attempted to train DL models to identify patients with hypertension [44,49,50]. The best result was reported by Zhang and colleagues using a cross-sectional Chinese dataset and neural network (NN) model [49]. Their model achieved an AUC of 0.77 in classifying patients with self-reported hypertension.

3.1.3. Hyperglycemia and Dyslipidemia

The overall performance of DL models in estimating outcomes associated with hyperglycemia and dyslipidemia using retinal images was not robust. For the fundus-based prediction of HbA1c, the MAE reported in different studies ranged between 0.33–1.39%, with a low R^2 of <0.10 in most studies [41,47,48]. Similar poor model performance and low R^2 were observed for most DL models trained to predict blood glucose level and lipid profile [47,48]. An exception was a model developed by Zhang et al., which was able to discriminate patients with self-reported hyperglycemia and dyslipidemia from normal controls with an AUC of 0.88 and 0.70, respectively [49].

3.1.4. Sex

Most DL studies predicting sex only performed internal validation, and in these studies, the models typically achieved an AUC of >0.95 during internal validation [41,47,48,51]. A notable exception was the study by Rim et al., in which the model was trained to predict multiple biomarkers, including sex. During external validation with 4 datasets obtained from patients of different ethnicities, this particular model predicting sex achieved an AUC ranging from 0.80 to 0.91 [47]. In the study by Korot et al., external validation was also performed using another local dataset, and their model achieved an accuracy of 78.6% [51].

3.1.5. Age

For retinal-image-based prediction of age, most studies reported similar MAEs in internal validation, ranging from 2.43 to 3.55 years [41,47,48,52]. Khan et al. also trained the DL model to predict age > 70 years and reported an AUC of 0.90 for this task [44]. Interestingly, Zu et al. further calculated the retinal age gap, which was the difference between chronological age and the age predicted by DL [52]. Using mortality data in the national EHR, they found that each 1-year increase in the retinal age gap was associated with a 2% risk increase (hazard ratio [HR] = 1.02, p = 0.020) in all-cause mortality. This novel finding suggests DL-based retinal "age" may be a better marker for senescence on a tissue level than chronological age.

3.1.6. Other Systemic Biomarkers and Disease Status

Other systemic biomarkers examined in DL-based oculomics included ethnicity, medication use, body composition, systemic organ functions, hematological parameters, and smoking status. Khan et al.'s model predicted ethnicity (Hispanic/Latino, non-Hispanic/Latino, others) based on fundus photographs using EHR as the ground truth, and reached an AUC of 0.93 [44]. Their model also showed a modest ability (AUC = 0.78–0.82) in identifying patients who take specific class of medications, such as angiotensin II receptor blockers and angiotensin-converting enzyme (ACE) inhibitors. In the study by Mitani et al., the DL model was trained to predict hemoglobin (Hb) and anemia, defined as Hb < 12 g/dL for women and <13 g/dL for men based on guidelines from the World Health Organization (WHO), using three types of data: retinal fundus images, participant metadata (race/ethnicity, age, sex and BP), and the combination of retinal images and metadata (multimodal data) [53]. The multimodal training data yielded the best model performance, with an AUC of 0.88 for anemia prediction and an MAE of 0.63 g/dL for Hb estimation. In contrast, the model trained only with retinal images yielded an AUC of 0.74 for anemia prediction and an MAE of 0.73 g/dL for Hb estimation. For the prediction of self-reported smoking status using fundus photographs, past studies [41,44,48,49,54] have reported models with AUC ranging from 0.70 to 0.86. As for the prediction of body mass index (BMI), most studies reported an MAE within 2–4 kg/m^2 and a low R^2 < 0.30 [41,47,48].

Of note, Rim et al. reported an ambitious study that trained NN models to predict a total of 47 systemic biomarkers using retinal fundus photographs [47]. Although satisfactory results were achieved for sex (AUC = 0.96 in internal validation, AUC = 0.80–0.91 in external validation) and age (MAEs = 2.43 years in internal validation, MAEs = 3.4–4.5 years in external validation) prediction, the height prediction (MAEs = 5.5–7.1 cm), weight (MAEs = 8.3–11.8 kg), BMI (MAEs = 2.4–3.5 kg/m^2), and creatinine (MAEs = 0.11–0.17 mg/dL) showed limited accuracy and generalizability in external validation with datasets of other ethnicities (R^2 < 0.30 for all). Other biomarkers, such as C-reactive protein, thyroid functions, and blood cell counts, could not be predicted from retinal fundus images using DL in this study.

For chronic kidney disease (CKD) prediction, Sabanayagam et al. presented DL models that predicted the presence of CKD, defined as an estimated glomerular filtration rate (eGFR) < 60 mL/min per 1.73 m^2, via retinal image analysis [55]. In their study,

3 model variations were trained: using only retinal fundus images, using only selected clinical data, and using both retinal images and clinical data (multimodal data). An AUC ranging from 0.73–0.84 and 0.81–0.86 was achieved for the retinal-image-only model and the multimodal data model, respectively, in external validation. Zhang et al. [56] presented a similar study that used 3 DL model variations to predict CKD. In external validation, an AUC ranging from 0.87–0.89 and 0.88–0.90 was reported for the retinal-image-only model and the multimodal data model, respectively. Additional analysis was performed to predict the eGFR values based on fundus photographs, and the DL models achieved an MAE ranging from 11–13 mL/min per 1.73 m^2 (R^2: 0.33–0.48) in external validation [56].

Tian et al. used retinal fundus images and DL techniques to predict the presence of Alzheimer's Disease (AD) [57]. Patients diagnosed with AD were identified based on ICD codes in the EHR. The authors used DL techniques to segment retinal vessels, and then the segmentation maps were used for classification via a support vector machine (SVM). An overall accuracy of 82% (sensitivity: 0.79%, specificity: 0.85%) for discriminating normal subjects from subjects with AD was achieved. Saliency map analysis demonstrated that small retinal vessels were more prominently activated than large retinal vessels during decision making.

3.2. Optical Coherence Tomography

3.2.1. Multiple Sclerosis (MS)

Compare to color fundus photographs, OCT is less commonly used in DL-based oculomics. Of the DL-based oculomics studies involving OCT, MS is the most studied systemic condition. In the study by Montolío et al., the performances of different ML algorithms, including linear regression, SVM, decision tree, k-nearest neighbors, Naïve Bayes, ensemble classifier and long short-term memory recurrent NN, in diagnosing MS and predicting the long-term disability course of MS were compared [58]. The diagnosis of MS was extracted from EHR and based on standard clinical and neuroimaging criteria (the McDonald criteria), [59] and the long-term disability ground truth was based on the expanded disability status scale (EDSS) scoring. All the ML models were trained with both clinical data and OCT-measured retinal nerve fiber layer (RNFL) thickness. The ensemble classifier, which performs prediction based on the weighted votes by various individual classifiers, [60] showed the best results for diagnosing MS (accuracy = 88%, AUC = 0.88), while the recurrent NN model showed the best prediction of long-term disability (accuracy = 82%, AUC = 0.82). In another study by López-Dorado et al., an NN model was also trained to diagnose MS using OCT images, with the ground truth determined by a neurologist based on the McDonald criteria [61]. Their model achieved a diagnostic accuracy of >90%. Additionally, they found the OCT-measured ganglion cell layer and whole retinal thicknesses to be the most discriminative features for diagnosing MS.

3.2.2. Age and Sex

Using OCT images centered on the optic nerve head and fovea, the MAE of DL-based age prediction ranged between 3.3–6 years, [62–65] with the best result reported by Hassan et al. [65]. Notably, in the study by Shigueoka et al., the CNN model revealed different correlations between the different retinal layers and age, [62] but this finding was not replicated in the study by Chueh et al. [64]. As for the OCT-based prediction of sex, accuracies and AUC ranged from 68% to 86% [63–65]. One study further compared the performances of DL models predicting sex using OCT foveal contour, OCT macular thickness, and infrared fundus photography, and showed the OCT foveal contour was most predictive [64].

Generally, as compared to color fundus photograph studies, OCT studies produced less robust DL models in predicting systemic biomarkers. Furthermore, most published OCT studies lacked external, independent validations.

4. Conclusions and Future Direction

Most of the published studies to date only used a single imaging modality, e.g., either color fundus photograph or OCT, for model training. Ideally, multiple imaging modalities should be used simultaneously for model training. For example, in a recent study published in 2022 by Wisely et al., multimodal retinal imaging consisting of OCT, OCT angiography, and ultra-widefield pseudo-color and ultra-widefield autofluorescence images were used to train a CNN model in predicting symptomatic AD [66]. In addition to multimodal retinal imaging, tabular clinical data can also be incorporated into model training. For example, in the studies by Sabanayagam et al. and Zhang et al., incorporating relevant demographic data such as age, gender, ethnicity, etc. were found to improve the prediction of CKD from color fundus photographs [55,56]. However, the incorporation of multimodal retinal imaging and different data types into model training will inevitably increase the technical complexity from a machine learning point of view. "Detailed analysis of salient retinal regions/features associated with DL predictability will provide further insights into ocular-systemic relationships. Such information was only provided by a limited number of studies included in this review, most of which used DL to predict age, sex and CVD via color fundus images (Table 1). For future directions, it remains to be seen how these deep learning-based oculomics models will be incorporated into clinical care and whether management decisions influenced by these models will lead to improved clinical outcomes.

Table 1. Salient retinal fundus regions/features associated with deep learning predictions.

Study, Publication Year (Country)	Prediction Targets	Salient Regions/Features Identified
Cardiovascular diseases (CVD) and CVD risk factors		
Poplin et al. 2018 [41] (United States of America [USA])	5-year major adverse cardiovascular events	Retinal vessels (for major CVD risk factors)
Chang et al., 2020 [42] (Korea)	Carotid artery atherosclerosis	Optic disc and retinal vessels
Son et al., 2020 [43] (Korea)	Accumulation of coronary artery calcium	Central main retinal vessel branches
Age		
	Age	Retinal vessels
		Optic disc and retinal vessels
Zhu et al. 2022 [53] (China)		Peri-vascular regions
Sex		
Poplin et al. 2018 [41] (USA)		Optic disc and retinal vessels
Rim et al. 2020 [47] (Singapore)	Sex	Optic disc and retinal vessels
Korot et al. 2021 [51] (United Kingdom)		Fovea, optic nerve and vascular arcades

Author Contributions: Study conception and design: J.-H.W. and T.Y.A.L. Literature search and data collection: J.-H.W. Analysis and interpretation of data: J.-H.W. and T.Y.A.L. Drafting of the manuscript: J.-H.W. and T.Y.A.L. Critical revision of the manuscript: J.-H.W. and T.Y.A.L. Supervision of study conduction: T.Y.A.L. Approval of the final version for submission: J.-H.W. and T.Y.A.L. All authors have read and agreed to the published version of the manuscript.

Funding: This research received no external funding.

Institutional Review Board Statement: Not applicable.

Informed Consent Statement: Not applicable.

Data Availability Statement: Not applicable.

Conflicts of Interest: The authors declare no conflict of interest.

References

1. Wagner, S.K.; Fu, D.J.; Faes, L.; Liu, X.; Huemer, J.; Khalid, H.; Ferraz, D.; Korot, E.; Kelly, C.; Balaskas, K.; et al. Insights into Systemic Disease through Retinal Imaging-Based Oculomics. *Transl. Vis. Sci. Technol.* **2020**, *9*, 6. [CrossRef] [PubMed]
2. Gupta, K.; Reddy, S. Heart, Eye, and Artificial Intelligence: A Review. *Cardiol. Res.* **2021**, *12*, 132–139. [CrossRef] [PubMed]
3. Vujosevic, S.; Parra, M.M.; Hartnett, M.E.; O'Toole, L.; Nuzzi, A.; Limoli, C.; Villani, E.; Nucci, P. Optical coherence tomography as retinal imaging biomarker of neuroinflammation/neurodegeneration in systemic disorders in adults and children. *Eye* **2022**. [CrossRef]
4. MacGillivray, T.J.; Trucco, E.; Cameron, J.R.; Dhillon, B.; Houston, J.G.; van Beek, E.J. Retinal imaging as a source of biomarkers for diagnosis, characterization and prognosis of chronic illness or long-term conditions. *Br. J. Radiol.* **2014**, *87*, 20130832. [CrossRef]
5. London, A.; Benhar, I.; Schwartz, M. The retina as a window to the brain—From eye research to CNS disorders. *Nat. Rev. Neurol.* **2013**, *9*, 44–53. [CrossRef]
6. Country, M.W. Retinal metabolism: A comparative look at energetics in the retina. *Brain Res.* **2017**, *1672*, 50–57. [CrossRef]
7. Honavar, S.G. Oculomics—The eyes talk a great deal. *Indian J. Ophthalmol.* **2022**, *70*, 713. [CrossRef]
8. Fujimoto, J.G.; Pitris, C.; Boppart, S.A.; Brezinski, M.E. Optical coherence tomography: An emerging technology for biomedical imaging and optical biopsy. *Neoplasia* **2000**, *2*, 9–25. [CrossRef]
9. Bille, J.F. (Ed.) *High Resolution Imaging in Microscopy and Ophthalmology: New Frontiers in Biomedical Optics*; Springer: Cham, Switzerland, 2019.
10. Snyder, P.J.; Alber, J.; Alt, C.; Bain, L.J.; Bouma, B.E.; Bouwman, F.H.; DeBuc, D.C.; Campbell, M.C.W.; Carrillo, M.C.; Chew, E.Y.; et al. Retinal imaging in Alzheimer's and neurodegenerative diseases. *Alzheimer's Dement.* **2021**, *17*, 103–111. [CrossRef]
11. Christinaki, E.; Kulenovic, H.; Hadoux, X.; Baldassini, N.; Van Eijgen, J.; De Groef, L.; Stalmans, I.; van Wijngaarden, P. Retinal imaging biomarkers of neurodegenerative diseases. *Clin. Exp. Optom.* **2022**, *105*, 194–204. [CrossRef]
12. Owen, C.G.; Rudnicka, A.R.; Welikala, R.A.; Fraz, M.M.; Barman, S.A.; Luben, R.; Hayat, S.A.; Khaw, K.T.; Strachan, D.P.; Whincup, P.H.; et al. Retinal Vasculometry Associations with Cardiometabolic Risk Factors in the European Prospective Investigation of Cancer-Norfolk Study. *Ophthalmology* **2019**, *126*, 96–106. [CrossRef] [PubMed]
13. Liew, G.; Mitchell, P.; Rochtchina, E.; Wong, T.Y.; Hsu, W.; Lee, M.L.; Wainwright, A.; Wang, J.J. Fractal analysis of retinal microvasculature and coronary heart disease mortality. *Eur. Heart J.* **2010**, *32*, 422–429. [CrossRef] [PubMed]
14. Witt, N.; Wong, T.Y.; Hughes, A.D.; Chaturvedi, N.; Klein, B.E.; Evans, R.; McNamara, M.; Thom, S.A.M.; Klein, R. Abnormalities of Retinal Microvascular Structure and Risk of Mortality from Ischemic Heart Disease and Stroke. *Hypertension* **2006**, *47*, 975–981. [CrossRef] [PubMed]
15. McGeechan, K.; Liew, G.; Macaskill, P.; Irwig, L.; Klein, R.; Klein, B.E.; Wang, J.J.; Mitchell, P.; Vingerling, J.R.; Dejong, P.T.; et al. Meta-analysis: Retinal vessel caliber and risk for coronary heart disease. *Ann. Intern. Med.* **2009**, *151*, 404–413. [CrossRef] [PubMed]
16. McGeechan, K.; Liew, G.; Macaskill, P.; Irwig, L.; Klein, R.; Klein, B.E.; Wang, J.J.; Mitchell, P.; Vingerling, J.R.; de Jong, P.T.; et al. Prediction of incident stroke events based on retinal vessel caliber: A systematic review and individual-participant meta-analysis. *Am. J. Epidemiol.* **2009**, *170*, 1323–1332. [CrossRef]
17. Wong, T.Y.; Klein, R.; Couper, D.J.; Cooper, L.S.; Shahar, E.; Hubbard, L.D.; Wofford, M.R.; Sharrett, A.R. Retinal microvascular abnormalities and incident stroke: The Atherosclerosis Risk in Communities Study. *Lancet* **2001**, *358*, 1134–1140. [CrossRef]
18. Wong, T.Y.; Klein, R.; Sharrett, A.R.; Manolio, T.A.; Hubbard, L.D.; Marino, E.K.; Kuller, L.; Burke, G.; Tracy, R.P.; Polak, J.F.; et al. The prevalence and risk factors of retinal microvascular abnormalities in older persons: The Cardiovascular Health Study. *Ophthalmology* **2003**, *110*, 658–666. [CrossRef]
19. Lim, L.S.; Cheung, C.Y.-l.; Sabanayagam, C.; Lim, S.C.; Tai, E.S.; Huang, L.; Wong, T.Y. Structural Changes in the Retinal Microvasculature and Renal Function. *Investig. Ophthalmol. Vis. Sci.* **2013**, *54*, 2970–2976. [CrossRef]
20. Liew, G.; Mitchell, P.; Wong, T.Y.; Wang, J.J. Retinal microvascular signs are associated with chronic kidney disease in persons with and without diabetes. *Kidney Blood Press. Res.* **2012**, *35*, 589–594. [CrossRef]
21. Lupton, S.J.; Chiu, C.L.; Hodgson, L.A.; Tooher, J.; Ogle, R.; Wong, T.Y.; Hennessy, A.; Lind, J.M. Changes in retinal microvascular caliber precede the clinical onset of preeclampsia. *Hypertension* **2013**, *62*, 899–904. [CrossRef]
22. Petzold, A.; de Boer, J.F.; Schippling, S.; Vermersch, P.; Kardon, R.; Green, A.; Calabresi, P.A.; Polman, C. Optical coherence tomography in multiple sclerosis: A systematic review and meta-analysis. *Lancet Neurol.* **2010**, *9*, 921–932. [CrossRef] [PubMed]
23. Britze, J.; Frederiksen, J.L. Optical coherence tomography in multiple sclerosis. *Eye* **2018**, *32*, 884–888. [CrossRef] [PubMed]
24. Paul, F.; Calabresi, P.A.; Barkhof, F.; Green, A.J.; Kardon, R.; Sastre-Garriga, J.; Schippling, S.; Vermersch, P.; Saidha, S.; Gerendas, B.S.; et al. Optical coherence tomography in multiple sclerosis: A 3-year prospective multicenter study. *Ann. Clin. Transl. Neurol.* **2021**, *8*, 2235–2251. [CrossRef] [PubMed]
25. Marziani, E.; Pomati, S.; Ramolfo, P.; Cigada, M.; Giani, A.; Mariani, C.; Staurenghi, G. Evaluation of Retinal Nerve Fiber Layer and Ganglion Cell Layer Thickness in Alzheimer's Disease Using Spectral-Domain Optical Coherence Tomography. *Investig. Ophthalmol. Vis. Sci.* **2013**, *54*, 5953–5958. [CrossRef] [PubMed]
26. Wang, M.; Zhu, Y.; Shi, Z.; Li, C.; Shen, Y. Meta-analysis of the relationship of peripheral retinal nerve fiber layer thickness to Alzheimer's disease and mild cognitive impairment. *Shanghai Arch. Psychiatry* **2015**, *27*, 263–279.

27. Lian, T.-H.; Jin, Z.; Qu, Y.-Z.; Guo, P.; Guan, H.-Y.; Zhang, W.-J.; Ding, D.-Y.; Li, D.-N.; Li, L.-X.; Wang, X.-M.; et al. The Relationship Between Retinal Nerve Fiber Layer Thickness and Clinical Symptoms of Alzheimer's Disease. *Front. Aging Neurosci.* **2021**, *12*, 584244. [CrossRef]
28. Ko, F.; Muthy, Z.A.; Gallacher, J.; Sudlow, C.; Rees, G.; Yang, Q.; Keane, P.A.; Petzold, A.; Khaw, P.T.; Reisman, C.; et al. Association of Retinal Nerve Fiber Layer Thinning With Current and Future Cognitive Decline: A Study Using Optical Coherence Tomography. *JAMA Neurol.* **2018**, *75*, 1198–1205. [CrossRef]
29. Mutlu, U.; Colijn, J.M.; Ikram, M.A.; Bonnemaijer, P.W.M.; Licher, S.; Wolters, F.J.; Tiemeier, H.; Koudstaal, P.J.; Klaver, C.C.W.; Ikram, M.K. Association of Retinal Neurodegeneration on Optical Coherence Tomography with Dementia: A Population-Based Study. *JAMA Neurol.* **2018**, *75*, 1256–1263. [CrossRef]
30. Chan, H.P.; Samala, R.K.; Hadjiiski, L.M.; Zhou, C. Deep Learning in Medical Image Analysis. *Adv. Exp. Med. Biol.* **2020**, *1213*, 3–21.
31. Shen, D.; Wu, G.; Suk, H.I. Deep Learning in Medical Image Analysis. *Annu. Rev. Biomed. Eng.* **2017**, *19*, 221–248. [CrossRef]
32. LeCun, Y.; Bengio, Y.; Hinton, G. Deep learning. *Nature* **2015**, *521*, 436–444. [CrossRef] [PubMed]
33. Wu, J.H.; Liu, T.Y.A.; Hsu, W.T.; Ho, J.H.; Lee, C.C. Performance and Limitation of Machine Learning Algorithms for Diabetic Retinopathy Screening: Meta-analysis. *J. Med. Internet Res.* **2021**, *23*, e23863. [CrossRef] [PubMed]
34. Abràmoff, M.D.; Lou, Y.; Erginay, A.; Clarida, W.; Amelon, R.; Folk, J.C.; Niemeijer, M. Improved Automated Detection of Diabetic Retinopathy on a Publicly Available Dataset Through Integration of Deep Learning. *Invest. Ophthalmol. Vis. Sci.* **2016**, *57*, 5200–5206. [CrossRef] [PubMed]
35. De Fauw, J.; Ledsam, J.R.; Romera-Paredes, B.; Nikolov, S.; Tomasev, N.; Blackwell, S.; Askham, H.; Glorot, X.; O'Donoghue, B.; Visentin, D.; et al. Clinically applicable deep learning for diagnosis and referral in retinal disease. *Nat. Med.* **2018**, *24*, 1342–1350. [CrossRef]
36. Lee, C.S.; Baughman, D.M.; Lee, A.Y. Deep Learning Is Effective for Classifying Normal versus Age-Related Macular Degeneration OCT Images. *Ophthalmol. Retin.* **2017**, *1*, 322–327. [CrossRef]
37. Gulshan, V.; Peng, L.; Coram, M.; Stumpe, M.C.; Wu, D.; Narayanaswamy, A.; Venugopalan, S.; Widner, K.; Madams, T.; Cuadros, J.; et al. Development and Validation of a Deep Learning Algorithm for Detection of Diabetic Retinopathy in Retinal Fundus Photographs. *JAMA* **2016**, *316*, 2402–2410. [CrossRef]
38. Grassmann, F.; Mengelkamp, J.; Brandl, C.; Harsch, S.; Zimmermann, M.E.; Linkohr, B.; Peters, A.; Heid, I.M.; Palm, C.; Weber, B.H.F. A Deep Learning Algorithm for Prediction of Age-Related Eye Disease Study Severity Scale for Age-Related Macular Degeneration from Color Fundus Photography. *Ophthalmology* **2018**, *125*, 1410–1420. [CrossRef]
39. Ting, D.S.W.; Cheung, C.Y.; Lim, G.; Tan, G.S.W.; Quang, N.D.; Gan, A.; Hamzah, H.; Garcia-Franco, R.; San Yeo, I.Y.; Lee, S.Y.; et al. Development and Validation of a Deep Learning System for Diabetic Retinopathy and Related Eye Diseases Using Retinal Images from Multiethnic Populations with Diabetes. *JAMA* **2017**, *318*, 2211–2223. [CrossRef]
40. Abràmoff, M.D.; Lavin, P.T.; Birch, M.; Shah, N.; Folk, J.C. Pivotal trial of an autonomous AI-based diagnostic system for detection of diabetic retinopathy in primary care offices. *npj Digit. Med.* **2018**, *1*, 39. [CrossRef]
41. Poplin, R.; Varadarajan, A.V.; Blumer, K.; Liu, Y.; McConnell, M.V.; Corrado, G.S.; Peng, L.; Webster, D.R. Prediction of cardiovascular risk factors from retinal fundus photographs via deep learning. *Nat. Biomed. Eng.* **2018**, *2*, 158–164. [CrossRef]
42. Chang, J.; Ko, A.; Park, S.M.; Choi, S.; Kim, K.; Kim, S.M.; Yun, J.M.; Kang, U.; Shin, I.H.; Shin, J.Y.; et al. Association of Cardiovascular Mortality and Deep Learning-Funduscopic Atherosclerosis Score derived from Retinal Fundus Images. *Am. J. Ophthalmol.* **2020**, *217*, 121–130. [CrossRef] [PubMed]
43. Son, J.; Shin, J.Y.; Chun, E.J.; Jung, K.-H.; Park, K.H.; Park, S.J. Predicting High Coronary Artery Calcium Score from Retinal Fundus Images With Deep Learning Algorithms. *Transl. Vis. Sci. Technol.* **2020**, *9*, 28. [CrossRef] [PubMed]
44. Khan, N.C.; Perera, C.; Dow, E.R.; Chen, K.M.; Mahajan, V.B.; Mruthyunjaya, P.; Do, D.V.; Leng, T.; Myung, D. Predicting Systemic Health Features from Retinal Fundus Images Using Transfer-Learning-Based Artificial Intelligence Models. *Diagnostics* **2022**, *12*, 1714. [CrossRef]
45. Cheung, C.Y.; Xu, D.; Cheng, C.-Y.; Sabanayagam, C.; Tham, Y.-C.; Yu, M.; Rim, T.H.; Chai, C.Y.; Gopinath, B.; Mitchell, P.; et al. A deep-learning system for the assessment of cardiovascular disease risk via the measurement of retinal-vessel calibre. *Nat. Biomed. Eng.* **2021**, *5*, 498–508. [CrossRef] [PubMed]
46. Ma, Y.; Xiong, J.; Zhu, Y.; Ge, Z.; Hua, R.; Fu, M.; Li, C.; Wang, B.; Dong, L.; Zhao, X.; et al. Development and validation of a deep learning algorithm using fundus photographs to predict 10-year risk of ischemic cardiovascular diseases among Chinese population. *medRxiv* **2021**. medRxiv:2021.04.15.21255176.
47. Rim, T.H.; Lee, G.; Kim, Y.; Tham, Y.C.; Lee, C.J.; Baik, S.J.; Kim, Y.A.; Yu, M.; Deshmukh, M.; Lee, B.K.; et al. Prediction of systemic biomarkers from retinal photographs: Development and validation of deep-learning algorithms. *Lancet Digit. Health* **2020**, *2*, e526–e536. [CrossRef]
48. Gerrits, N.; Elen, B.; Craenendonck, T.V.; Triantafyllidou, D.; Petropoulos, I.N.; Malik, R.A.; De Boever, P. Age and sex affect deep learning prediction of cardiometabolic risk factors from retinal images. *Sci. Rep.* **2020**, *10*, 9432. [CrossRef]
49. Zhang, L.; Yuan, M.; An, Z.; Zhao, X.; Wu, H.; Li, H.; Wang, Y.; Sun, B.; Li, H.; Ding, S.; et al. Prediction of hypertension, hyperglycemia and dyslipidemia from retinal fundus photographs via deep learning: A cross-sectional study of chronic diseases in central China. *PLoS ONE* **2020**, *15*, e0233166. [CrossRef] [PubMed]
50. Dai, G.; He, W.; Xu, L.; Pazo, E.E.; Lin, T.; Liu, S.; Zhang, C. Exploring the effect of hypertension on retinal microvasculature using deep learning on East Asian population. *PLoS ONE* **2020**, *15*, e0230111. [CrossRef]

51. Korot, E.; Pontikos, N.; Liu, X.; Wagner, S.K.; Faes, L.; Huemer, J.; Balaskas, K.; Denniston, A.K.; Khawaja, A.; Keane, P.A. Predicting sex from retinal fundus photographs using automated deep learning. *Sci. Rep.* **2021**, *11*, 10286. [CrossRef]
52. Zhu, Z.; Shi, D.; Guankai, P.; Tan, Z.; Shang, X.; Hu, W.; Liao, H.; Zhang, X.; Huang, Y.; Yu, H.; et al. Retinal age gap as a predictive biomarker for mortality risk. *Br. J. Ophthalmol.* **2022**. [CrossRef] [PubMed]
53. Mitani, A.; Huang, A.; Venugopalan, S.; Corrado, G.S.; Peng, L.; Webster, D.R.; Hammel, N.; Liu, Y.; Varadarajan, A.V. Detection of anaemia from retinal fundus images via deep learning. *Nat. Biomed. Eng.* **2020**, *4*, 18–27. [CrossRef] [PubMed]
54. Vaghefi, E.; Yang, S.; Hill, S.; Humphrey, G.; Walker, N.; Squirrell, D. Detection of smoking status from retinal images; a Convolutional Neural Network study. *Sci. Rep.* **2019**, *9*, 7180. [CrossRef] [PubMed]
55. Sabanayagam, C.; Xu, D.; Ting, D.S.W.; Nusinovici, S.; Banu, R.; Hamzah, H.; Lim, C.; Tham, Y.C.; Cheung, C.Y.; Tai, E.S.; et al. A deep learning algorithm to detect chronic kidney disease from retinal photographs in community-based populations. *Lancet Digit. Health* **2020**, *2*, e295–e302. [CrossRef]
56. Zhang, K.; Liu, X.; Xu, J.; Yuan, J.; Cai, W.; Chen, T.; Wang, K.; Gao, Y.; Nie, S.; Xu, X.; et al. Deep-learning models for the detection and incidence prediction of chronic kidney disease and type 2 diabetes from retinal fundus images. *Nat. Biomed. Eng.* **2021**, *5*, 533–545. [CrossRef]
57. Tian, J.; Smith, G.; Guo, H.; Liu, B.; Pan, Z.; Wang, Z.; Xiong, S.; Fang, R. Modular machine learning for Alzheimer's disease classification from retinal vasculature. *Sci. Rep.* **2021**, *11*, 238. [CrossRef]
58. Montolío, A.; Martín-Gallego, A.; Cegoñino, J.; Orduna, E.; Vilades, E.; Garcia-Martin, E.; Palomar, A.P.d. Machine learning in diagnosis and disability prediction of multiple sclerosis using optical coherence tomography. *Comput. Biol. Med.* **2021**, *133*, 104416. [CrossRef]
59. McDonald, W.I.; Compston, A.; Edan, G.; Goodkin, D.; Hartung, H.P.; Lublin, F.D.; McFarland, H.F.; Paty, D.W.; Polman, C.H.; Reingold, S.C. Recommended diagnostic criteria for multiple sclerosis: Guidelines from the International Panel on the diagnosis of multiple sclerosis. *Ann. Neurol. Off. J. Am. Neurol. Assoc. Child Neurol. Soc.* **2001**, *50*, 121–127. [CrossRef]
60. Dietterich, T.G. (Ed.) *Ensemble Methods in Machine Learning. Multiple Classifier Systems*; Springer: Berlin/Heidelberg, Germany, 2000.
61. López-Dorado, A.; Ortiz, M.; Satue, M.; Rodrigo, M.J.; Barea, R.; Sánchez-Morla, E.M.; Cavaliere, C.; Rodríguez-Ascariz, J.M.; Orduna-Hospital, E.; Boquete, L.; et al. Early Diagnosis of Multiple Sclerosis Using Swept-Source Optical Coherence Tomography and Convolutional Neural Networks Trained with Data Augmentation. *Sensors* **2022**, *22*, 167. [CrossRef]
62. Shigueoka, L.S.; Mariottoni, E.B.; Thompson, A.C.; Jammal, A.A.; Costa, V.P.; Medeiros, F.A. Predicting Age From Optical Coherence Tomography Scans With Deep Learning. *Transl. Vis. Sci. Technol.* **2021**, *10*, 12. [CrossRef]
63. Mendoza, L.; Christopher, M.; Brye, N.; Proudfoot, J.A.; Belghith, A.; Bowd, C.; Rezapour, J.; Fazio, M.A.; Goldbaum, M.H.; Weinreb, R.N.; et al. Deep Learning Predicts Demographic and Clinical Characteristics from Optic Nerve Head OCT Circle and Radial Scans. *Investig. Ophthalmol. Vis. Sci.* **2021**, *62*, 2120.
64. Chueh, K.-M.; Hsieh, Y.-T.; Chen, H.H.; Ma, I.H.; Huang, S.-L. Identification of Sex and Age from Macular Optical Coherence Tomography and Feature Analysis Using Deep Learning. *Am. J. Ophthalmol.* **2022**, *235*, 221–228. [CrossRef] [PubMed]
65. Hassan, O.N.; Menten, M.J.; Bogunovic, H.; Schmidt-Erfurth, U.; Lotery, A.; Rueckert, D. (Eds.) Deep Learning Prediction Of Age And Sex From Optical Coherence Tomography. In Proceedings of the 2021 IEEE 18th International Symposium on Biomedical Imaging (ISBI), Nice, France, 13–16 April 2021.
66. Wisely, C.E.; Wang, D.; Henao, R.; Grewal, D.S.; Thompson, A.C.; Robbins, C.B.; Yoon, S.P.; Soundararajan, S.; Polascik, B.W.; Burke, J.R.; et al. Convolutional neural network to identify symptomatic Alzheimer's disease using multimodal retinal imaging. *Br. J. Ophthalmol.* **2022**, *106*, 388–395. [CrossRef] [PubMed]

Disclaimer/Publisher's Note: The statements, opinions and data contained in all publications are solely those of the individual author(s) and contributor(s) and not of MDPI and/or the editor(s). MDPI and/or the editor(s) disclaim responsibility for any injury to people or property resulting from any ideas, methods, instructions or products referred to in the content.

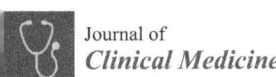

Case Report

Bilateral Branch Retinal Vein Occlusion after mRNA-SARS-CoV-2 Booster Dose Vaccination

Matteo Gironi [1,2,†], Rossella D'Aloisio [2,*,†], Tommaso Verdina [1], Benjamin Shkurko [3], Lisa Toto [2] and Rodolfo Mastropasqua [2]

1 Ophthalmology Clinic, University of Modena and Reggio Emilia, Azienda Ospedaliero-Universitaria di Modena, 41125 Policlinico, Italy
2 Ophthalmology Clinic, Department of Medicine and Science of Ageing, University G. D'Annunzio Chieti-Pescara, 66100 Chieti, Italy
3 Ophthalmology Clinic, Department of Medicine and Surgery, University of Parma, 43121 Parma, Italy
* Correspondence: ross.daloisio@gmail.com
† These authors contributed equally to the paper and should be considered as co-first authors.

Abstract: Purpose: We report a case of a patient with a bilateral branch retinal vein occlusion (BRVO) 24 h after a booster vaccination with the mRNA-1237 vaccine. Observations: Fluorescein angiography, performed at three weeks follow-up, showed vascular leakage and blockage, corresponding to hemorrhage areas associated with ischemic areas in the macula and along the arcades involved in the occlusion. Conclusions: The patient was scheduled for urgent injections of intravitreal ranibizumab and laser photocoagulation of the ischemic areas. To the best of our knowledge, this is the first case described of concomitant bilateral RVO after COVID-19 vaccination. The rapid onset of the side effects in a patient with multiple risk factors for thrombotic events suggests that vulnerable microvascular conditions require detailed investigations before administration of a COVID-19 vaccine.

Keywords: COVID; SARS-CoV-2; retinal vein occlusion; RVO; vaccination; branch retinal vein occlusion

1. Introduction

Vaccines are essential to limit the social impact of the COVID-19 pandemic. By January 2022, more than 9.5 billion doses of COVID-19 vaccines were administered worldwide.

Vaccine-related serious side effects reported in the literature have varied and have included cerebral venous sinus thrombosis and immune thrombotic thrombocytopenia [1]. Several types of ocular manifestations have also been reported [2].

To the best of our knowledge, no report on simultaneous bilateral retinal vein occlusion (RVO) consequent to vaccination has been described until now. Here, we report a case of a bilateral branch retinal vein occlusion (BRVO) after a booster vaccination with the mRNA-1237 vaccine (Moderna).

2. Case Report

A 50-year-old Caucasian man was referred to our Ophthalmological Emergency Service for painless sudden vision loss in both eyes, onset 24 h after a booster dose with the mRNA-1237 vaccine. He had received the mRNA-vaccine BNT162b2 for the first two vaccination doses, without side effects. No previous infection of SARS-CoV-2 was reported. Past medical history included an emergency hospitalization in 2020 for mild acute heart failure (NYHA II) in newly diagnosed dilated cardiomyopathy and arterial hypertension. At discharge, a multi-pharmacological antihypertensive treatment was set. A family history of heart attack was reported (father died at 50 of myocardial infarction). The patient is a non-smoker with mild obesity (BMI = 33.4).

During the ophthalmological evaluation, the patient was in treatment with Valproate and Lurasidone for psychotic syndrome. The latest previous blood tests did not show

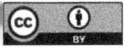

pathologically altered values, while the ECG revealed a modest alteration due to ventricular overload.

The ophthalmic evaluation revealed a best-corrected visual acuity of 20/200 in the right eye and 20/28 in the left eye. Intraocular pressure and anterior segment exams were normal in both eyes. A fundus examination showed congested tortuous veins associated with flame hemorrhages and cotton wool spots of superior-temporal arcade in the right eye and inferior-temporal arcade in the left eye. Pathological signs were more extensive in the right eye than in the left eye. (Figure 1A,B). High-resolution optical coherence tomography, performed at presentation, revealed significant macular edema in both eyes, as shows Figure 1.

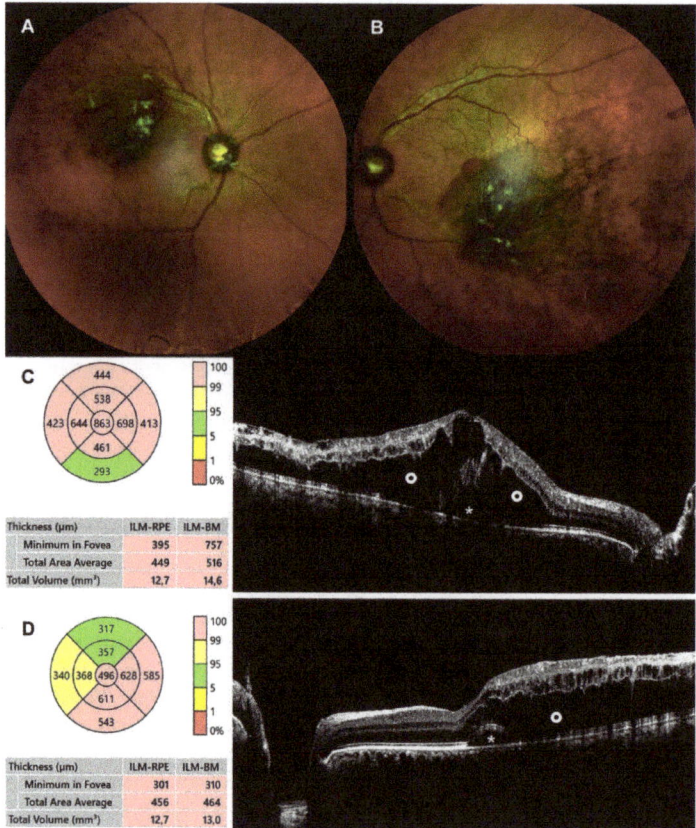

Figure 1. Baseline posterior pole multicolor image and optical coherence tomography of both eyes: (**top**) Fundus photographs showing widespread hemorrhages and axonal congestion upstream of the venous occlusion of superotemporal branch vein in the right eye (**A**) and inferotemporal branch vein in the left eye (**B**); (**bottom**) OCT macula (Macula 3D mode) shows a significant cystoid macular edema and intraretinal fluid (O), associated with subfoveal neuroretinal detachment (*) in both eyes, with a central macular thickness of 863 μm for the right eye (**C**) and 496 μm for the left eye (**D**).

The last previous eye examination was 6 months before vaccination, and it reported a retinal vascular tree within the age range, with no other relevant alterations.

Extensive screening blood examinations, including full blood cell counts and differential with peripheral blood smear, platelet count, electrolytes, lipid profile, fasting glycemia, iron tests, liver enzymes, serum protein, lipid profile, serum bilirubin, and serum creatinine, revealed only a mild alteration of liver functionalities. C-reactive protein was 0.3 mg/L (range 0–0.7) and erythrocyte sedimentation rate was 3 mm/h (range 2–28). Other screening blood examinations were performed, including thyroid hormones, vitamin B12, folate, serum homocysteine, glycated hemoglobin (HbA1c), anti-cardiolipin antibodies, thrombophilia screen, treponema pallidum screening, cytomegalovirus IgM-IgG, and serum HIV, which were all unremarkable.

Fluorescein angiography, performed at three weeks follow-up, showed vascular leakage and blockage, corresponding to the hemorrhage areas associated with ischemic areas in the macula and along the arcades involved in the occlusion (Figure 2).

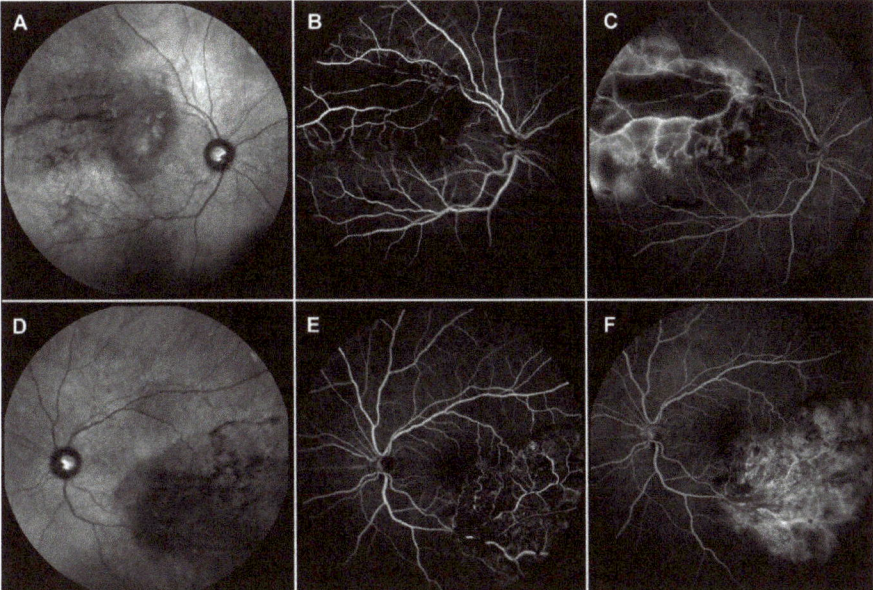

Figure 2. Fundus autofluorescence (FAF) and fluorescein angiography (FA) of both eyes at three weeks follow-up. FAF of the right (**A**) and left (**D**) eyes hyper-autofluorescence corresponding to intraretinal fluid near the fovea and hypo-autofluorescence as a result of blockage intraretinal hemorrhage. FA shows ischemic branch retinal vein occlusion with blockage corresponding to the retinal hemorrhage in early phases ((**B**), right and (**E**), left). Late phases showed extensive leakage in the area of branch retinal vein occlusion and clinically significant macular edema ((**C**), right and (**F**), left). Arm-retina time, 16 s; Right eye arteriovenous transit time, 42 s; Left eye arteriovenous transit time, 32 s.

The patient was scheduled for urgent injections of intravitreal ranibizumab and laser photocoagulation of ischemic areas.

3. Discussion

BRVO is the second most common retinal vascular disease. Despite this, the occurrence of concurrent bilateral BRVO is uncommon.

Here, we reported a case of bilateral BRVO likely due to booster dose vaccination. To the best of our knowledge, this is the first case described of concomitant bilateral RVO after COVID-19 vaccination.

Undoubtedly, our patient presented underlying conditions that moderately exacerbated thrombogenicity, such as hypertension and obesity, even if his blood cell counts and hemostasis tests were unremarkable [3].

In the literature, a few case reports of unilateral RVO after COVID-19 vaccination have been reported [2–5]. Nonetheless, one of these depicted a concomitant central retinal artery and vein occlusion after the second dose [6].

Recently, two case series on ocular complications after SARS-CoV-2 vaccination have shown that more than 50% of eyes who developed RVO had received an mRNA vaccine. The median time between vaccination and symptom exacerbation was 2 days [2,4]. No bilateral cases were identified in these series.

A case report of bilateral branch retinal vein occlusions secondary to sodium valproate therapy has been reported in the literature [7]. Sodium valproate can induce increased levels of serum homocysteine (HC), which is an independent factor for vascular events [8]. Despite this, the HC levels detected in the patient were within the range of normality (9 µmol/L).

Although the pathogenesis mechanism requires further study, possible hypotheses on such an adverse event are focusing on spike proteins as triggering an atypical procoagulant and proinflammatory response, especially in eyes more vulnerable to microvascular dysfunction [4].

4. Conclusions

In conclusion, here, we report a case where a drug-related vascular event relationship is very strong, because of concomitant manifestation in both eyes. The rapid onset of the side effects in a patient with multiple risk factors for thrombotic events suggests that vulnerable microvascular conditions require detailed investigations before administration of a COVID-19 vaccine.

Author Contributions: R.M., R.D., L.T. and M.G. wrote and revised the manuscript; T.V. and B.S. collected data and performed the clinical evaluation. All authors have read and agreed to the published version of the manuscript.

Funding: This research received no external funding.

Institutional Review Board Statement: The study was conducted in accordance with the Declaration of Helsinki and approved by the Institutional Review Board (Department of Medicine and Science of Ageing) of University of G.d'Annunzio Chieti-Pescara.

Informed Consent Statement: Written consent to publish this case report has been obtained from the patient. This report does not contain any personal identifying information.

Data Availability Statement: All data are available on a reasonable request to the corresponding author.

Conflicts of Interest: The authors declare no conflict of interest.

References

1. Abbattista, M.; Martinelli, I.; Peyvandi, F. Comparison of adverse drug reactions among four COVID-19 vaccines in Europe using the EudraVigilance database: Thrombosis at unusual sites. *J. Thromb. Haemost.* **2021**, *19*, 2554–2558. [CrossRef]
2. Bolletta, E.; Iannetta, D.; Mastrofilippo, V.; De Simone, L.; Gozzi, F.; Croci, S.; Bonacini, M.; Belloni, L.; Zerbini, A.; Adani, C.; et al. Uveitis and Other Ocular Complications Following COVID-19 Vaccination. *J. Clin. Med.* **2021**, *10*, 5960. [CrossRef]
3. Hayreh, S.S.; Zimmerman, B.; McCarthy, M.J.; Podhajsky, P. Systemic diseases associated with various types of retinal vein occlusion. *Am. J. Ophthalmol.* **2001**, *131*, 61–77. [CrossRef]
4. Park, H.S.; Byun, Y.; Byeon, S.H.; Kim, S.S.; Kim, Y.J.; Lee, C.S. Retinal Hemorrhage after SARS-CoV-2 Vaccination. *J. Clin. Med.* **2021**, *10*, 5705. [CrossRef]
5. Sacconi, R.; Simona, F.; Forte, P.; Querques, G. Retinal Vein Occlusion Following Two Doses of mRNA-1237 (Moderna) Immunization for SARS-Cov-2: A Case Report. *Ophthalmol. Ther.* **2021**, *11*, 1–6. [CrossRef]
6. Ikegami, Y.; Numaga, J.; Okano, N.; Fukuda, S.; Yamamoto, H.; Terada, Y. Combined central retinal artery and vein occlusion shortly after mRNA-SARS-CoV-2 vaccination. *QJM* **2022**, *114*, 884–885. [CrossRef]

7. Hussain, R.N.; Banerjee, S. Presumed bilateral branch retinal vein occlusions secondary to antiepileptic agents. *Clin. Ophthalmol.* **2011**, *5*, 609–611. [CrossRef]
8. Kaplan, E.D. Association between homocyst(e)ine levels and risk of vascular events. *Drugs Today* **2003**, *39*, 175–192. [CrossRef]

Disclaimer/Publisher's Note: The statements, opinions and data contained in all publications are solely those of the individual author(s) and contributor(s) and not of MDPI and/or the editor(s). MDPI and/or the editor(s) disclaim responsibility for any injury to people or property resulting from any ideas, methods, instructions or products referred to in the content.

MDPI
St. Alban-Anlage 66
4052 Basel
Switzerland
www.mdpi.com

Journal of Clinical Medicine Editorial Office
E-mail: jcm@mdpi.com
www.mdpi.com/journal/jcm

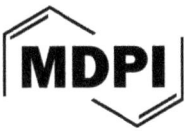

Disclaimer/Publisher's Note: The statements, opinions and data contained in all publications are solely those of the individual author(s) and contributor(s) and not of MDPI and/or the editor(s). MDPI and/or the editor(s) disclaim responsibility for any injury to people or property resulting from any ideas, methods, instructions or products referred to in the content.

www.ingramcontent.com/pod-product-compliance
Lightning Source LLC
LaVergne TN
LVHW070042120526
838202LV00101B/413